Written by Amber Rae Johnson
Illustrated by Felipe Reis

Urth Publishing

www.bigquestionsbooks.com

Facebook.com/bigquestionsbooks
Instagram.com/bigquestionsbooks
Twitter.com/BQbooks

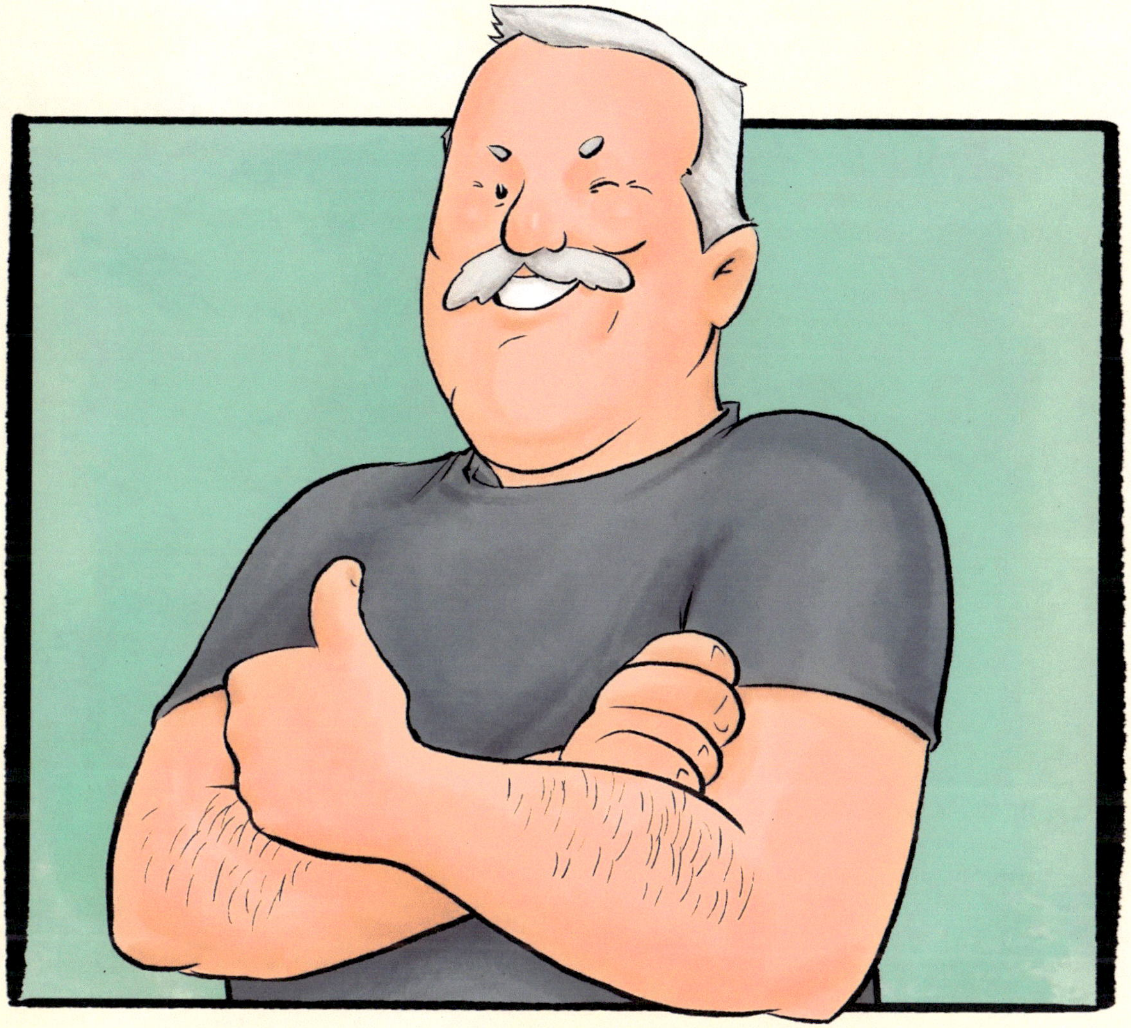

For my daddy, with humor and love, as he will never understand why I eat different food.

MAZE AND BALOO ARE CURIOUS BOYS, THINKING AND THINKING WHEN THEY PLAY WITH THEIR TOYS.

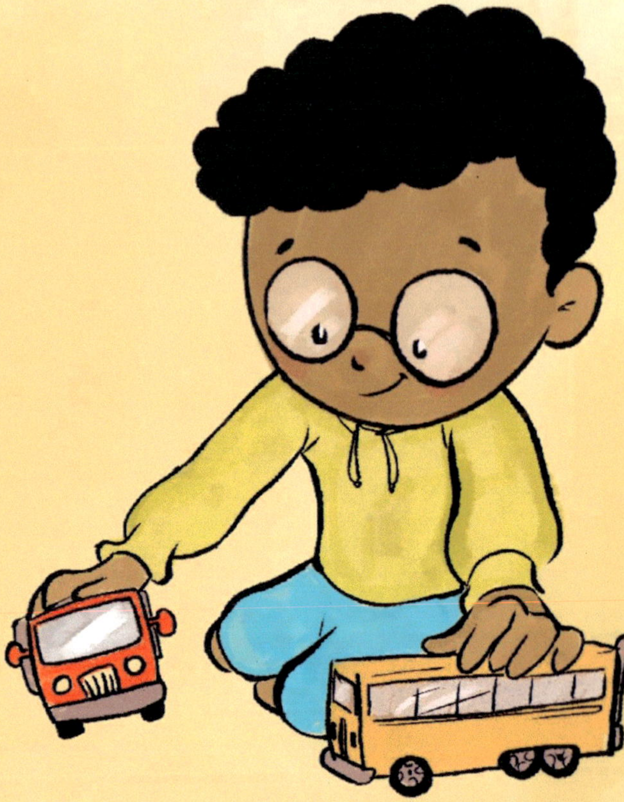

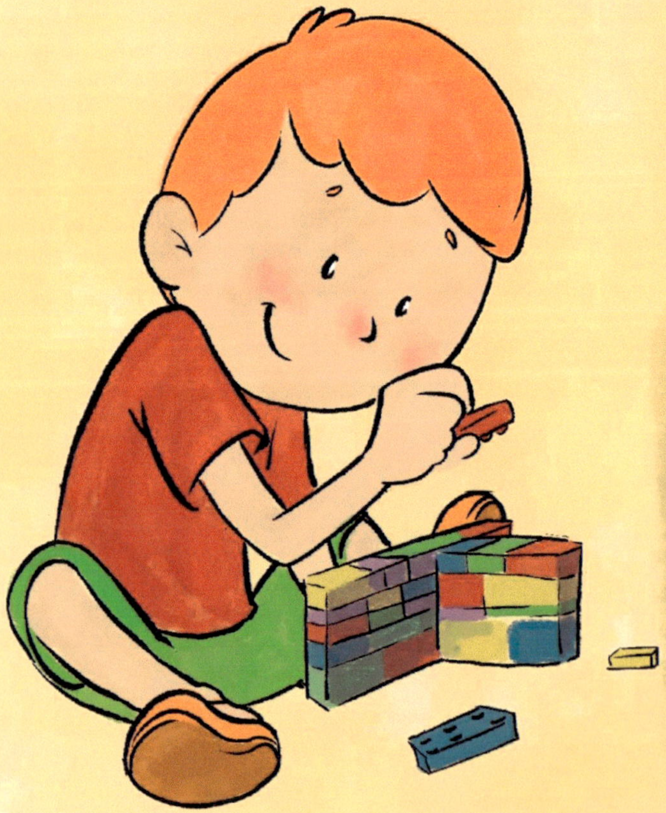

WHEN THEY HAVE BIG QUESTIONS THEY KNOW WHAT TO DO, THEY ASK SOMEONE SMART TO FIND OUT WHAT'S TRUE.

THEY RUN TO THEIR MOMS AND SIT ON THEIR LAPS AND PROMPT WHAT WILL BE ANOTHER BIG IMPORTANT CHAT.

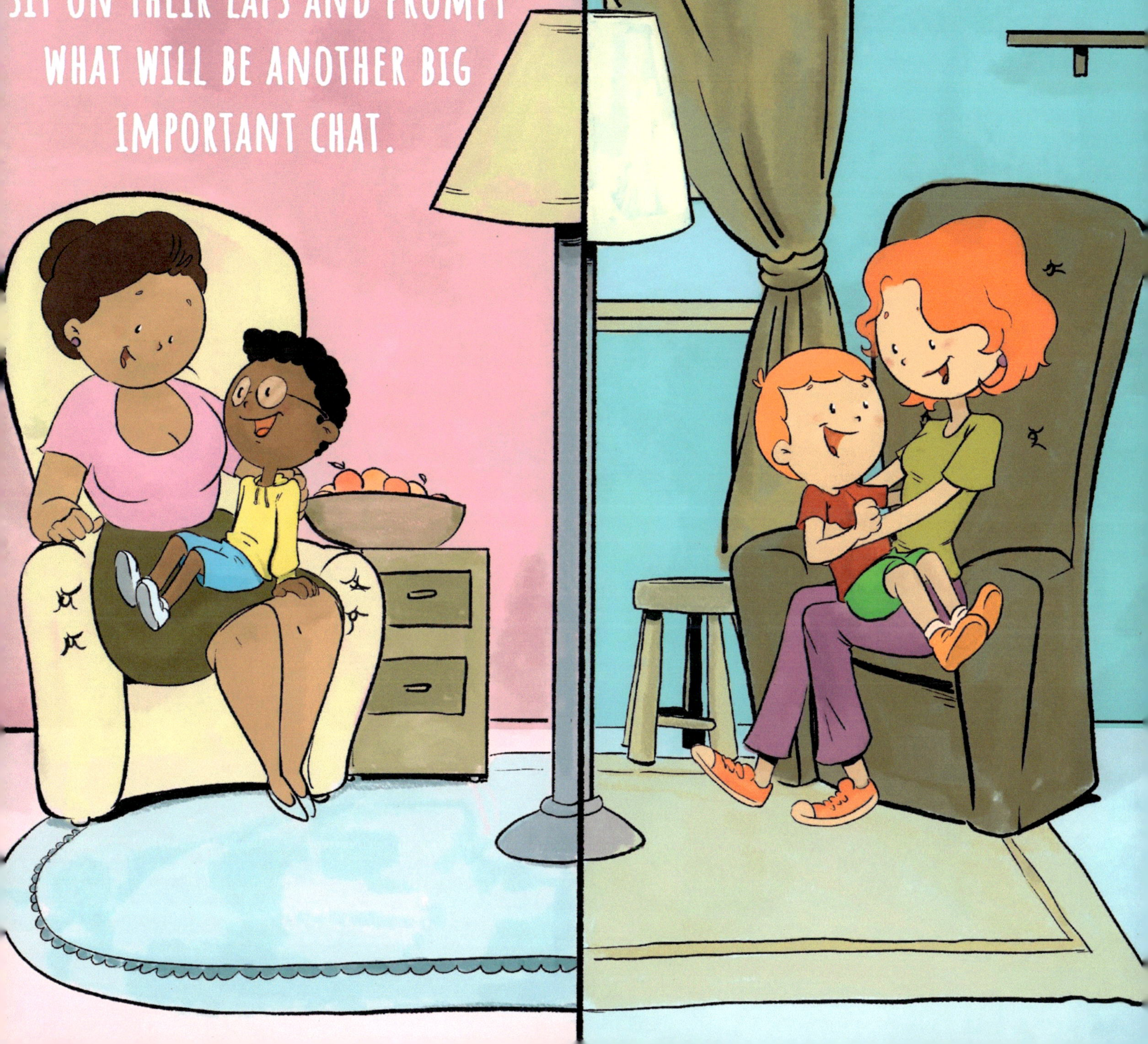

BIG QUESTIONS

WHY DO THEY EAT DIFFERENT FOOD?

WRITTEN BY
AMBER RAE JOHNSON

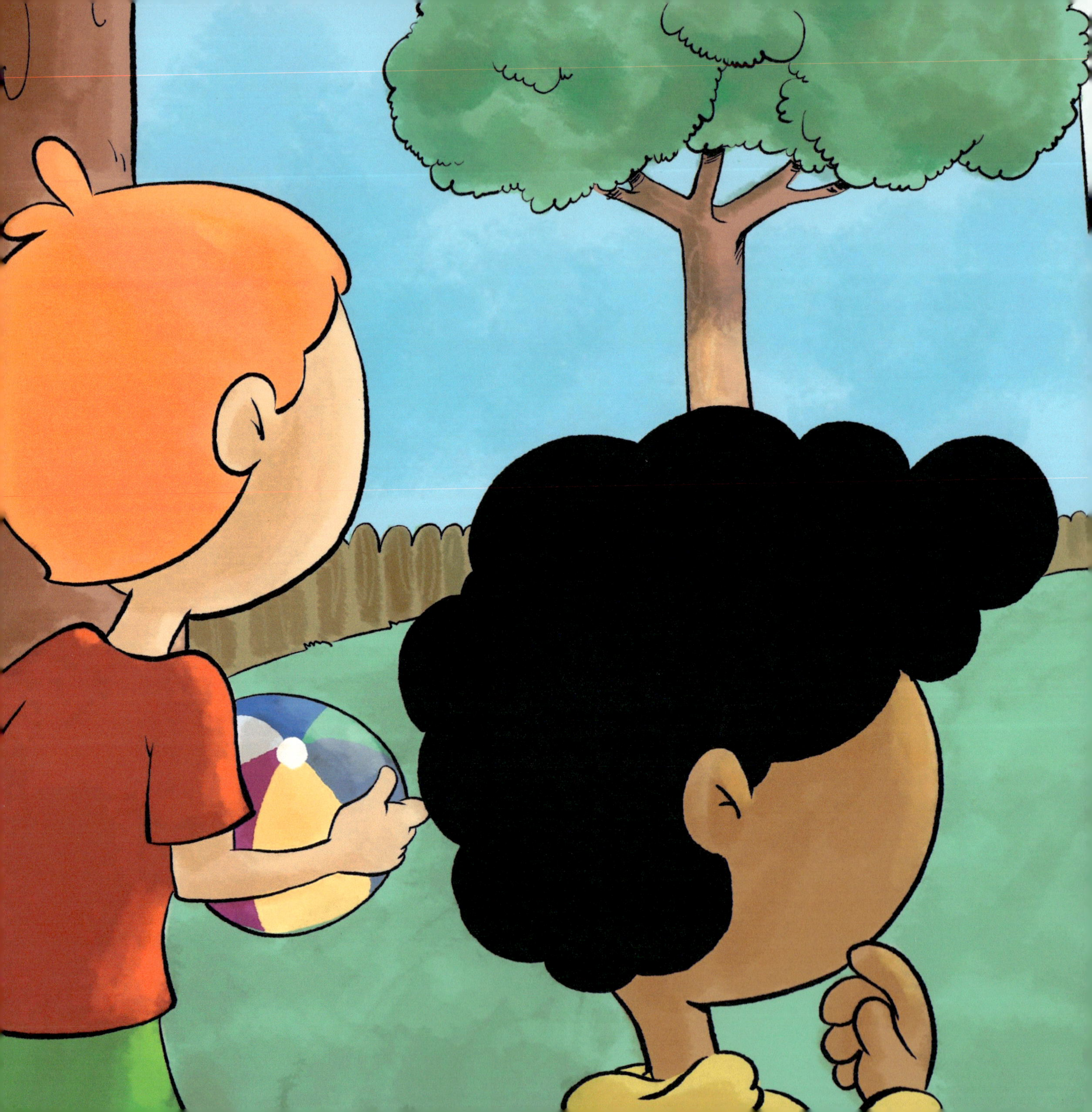

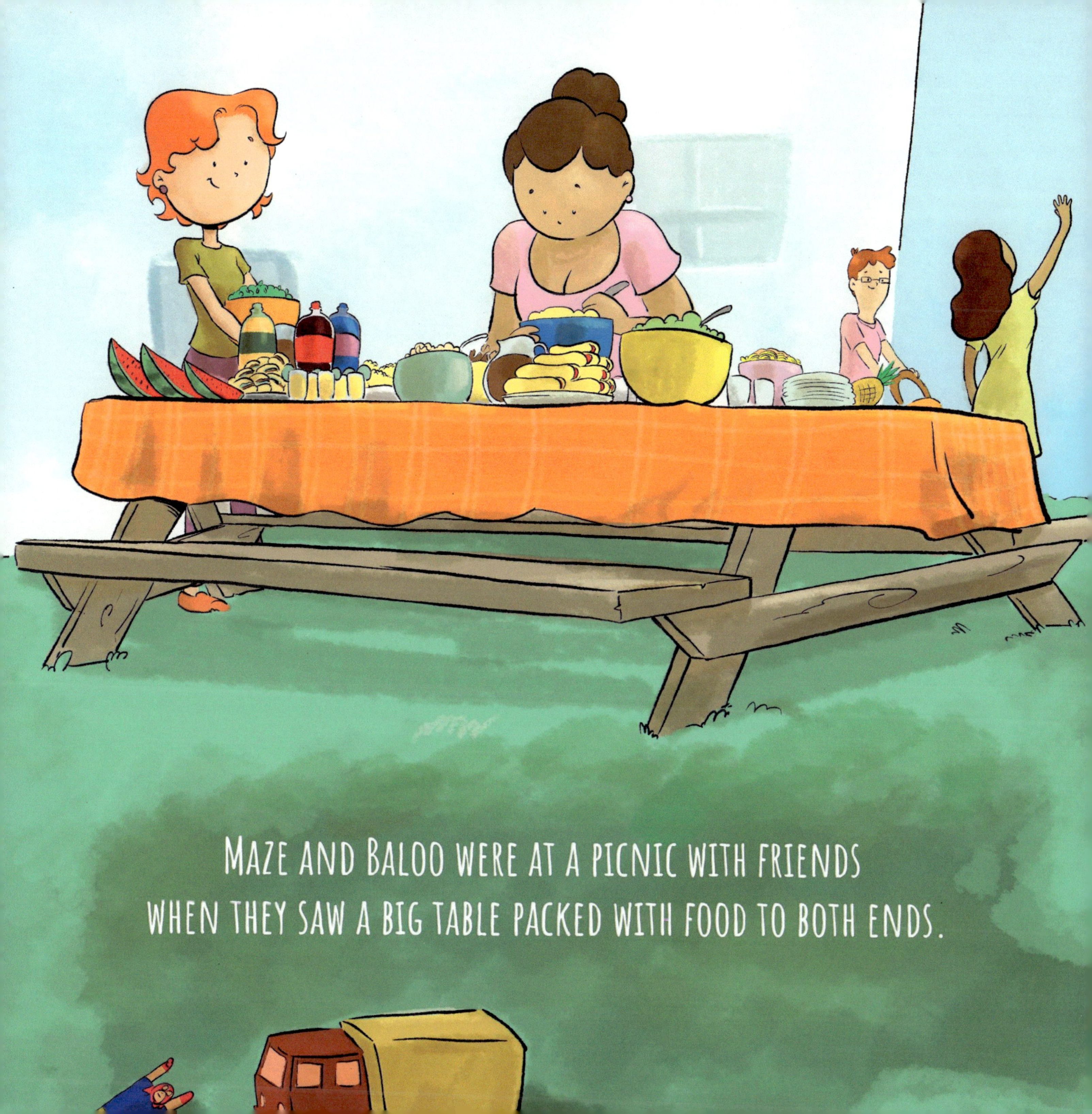

MAZE AND BALOO WERE AT A PICNIC WITH FRIENDS
WHEN THEY SAW A BIG TABLE PACKED WITH FOOD TO BOTH ENDS.

THERE WAS SO MUCH TO SEE AND WHILE THEIR MOMS MADE THEIR PLATES,
THEY COULDN'T HELP BUT NOTICE WHAT EVERYONE ATE.

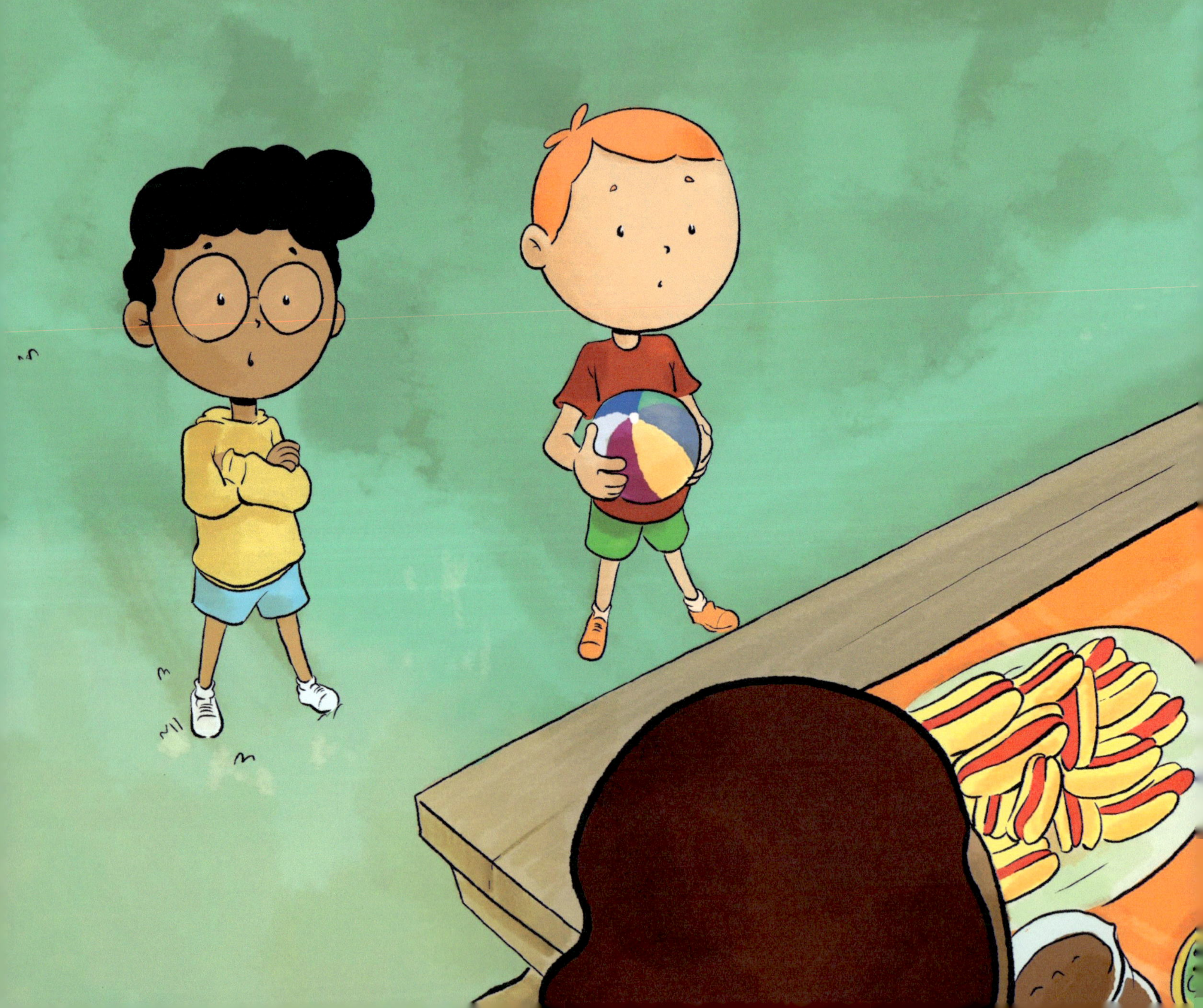

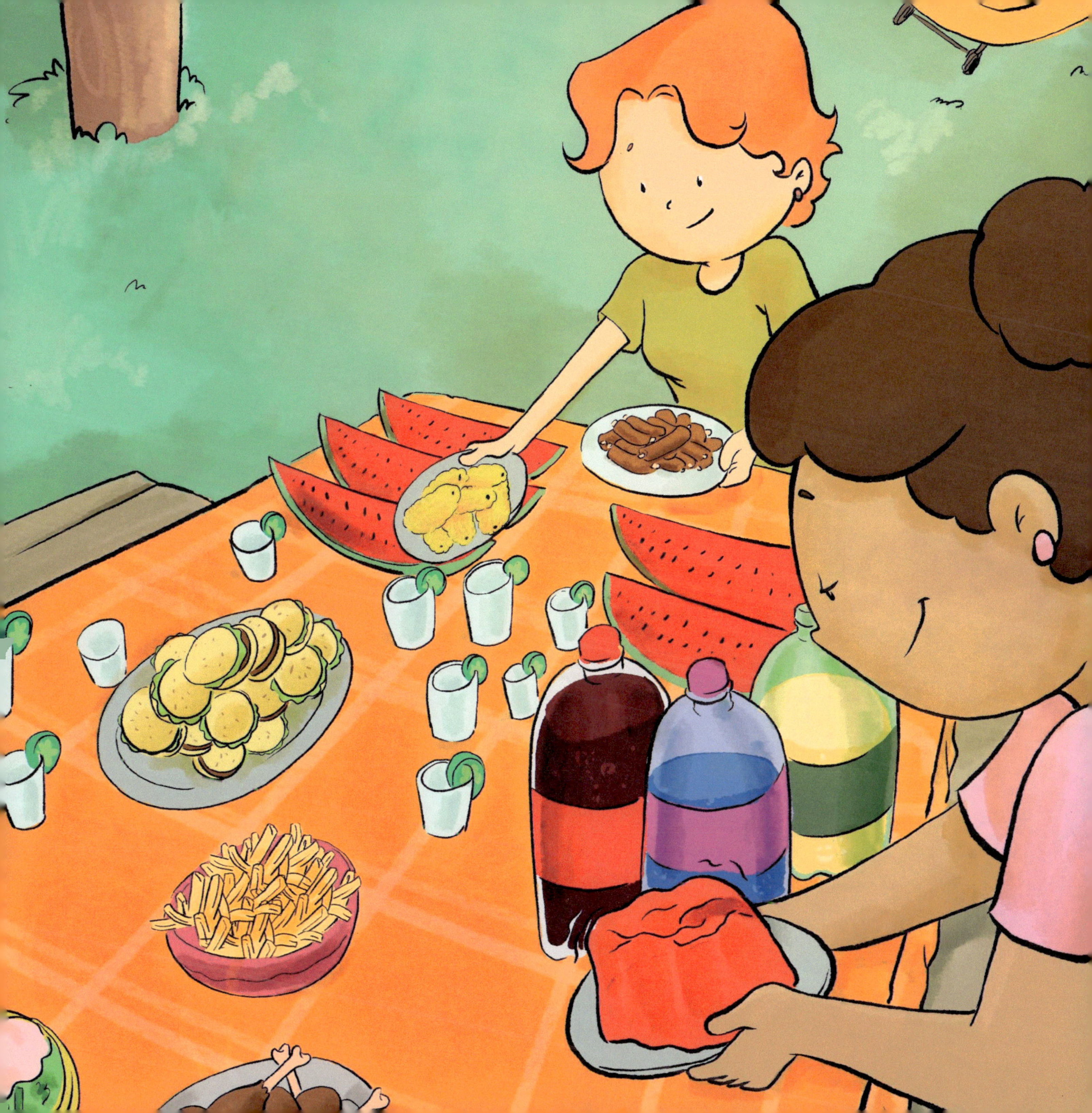

When they sat down to eat they saw many bright colors.
Their meals were full of only veggies and beans, unlike the others.

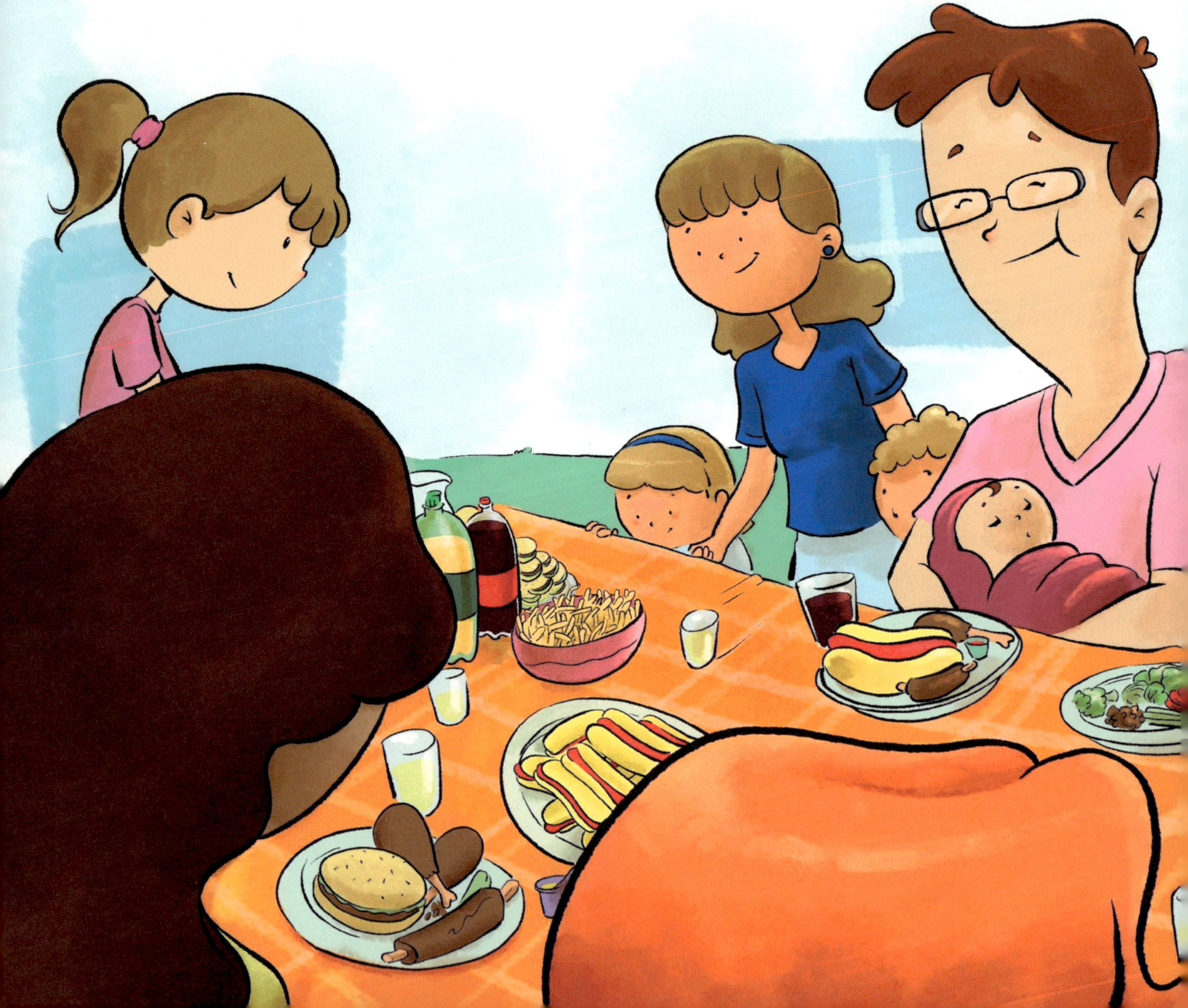

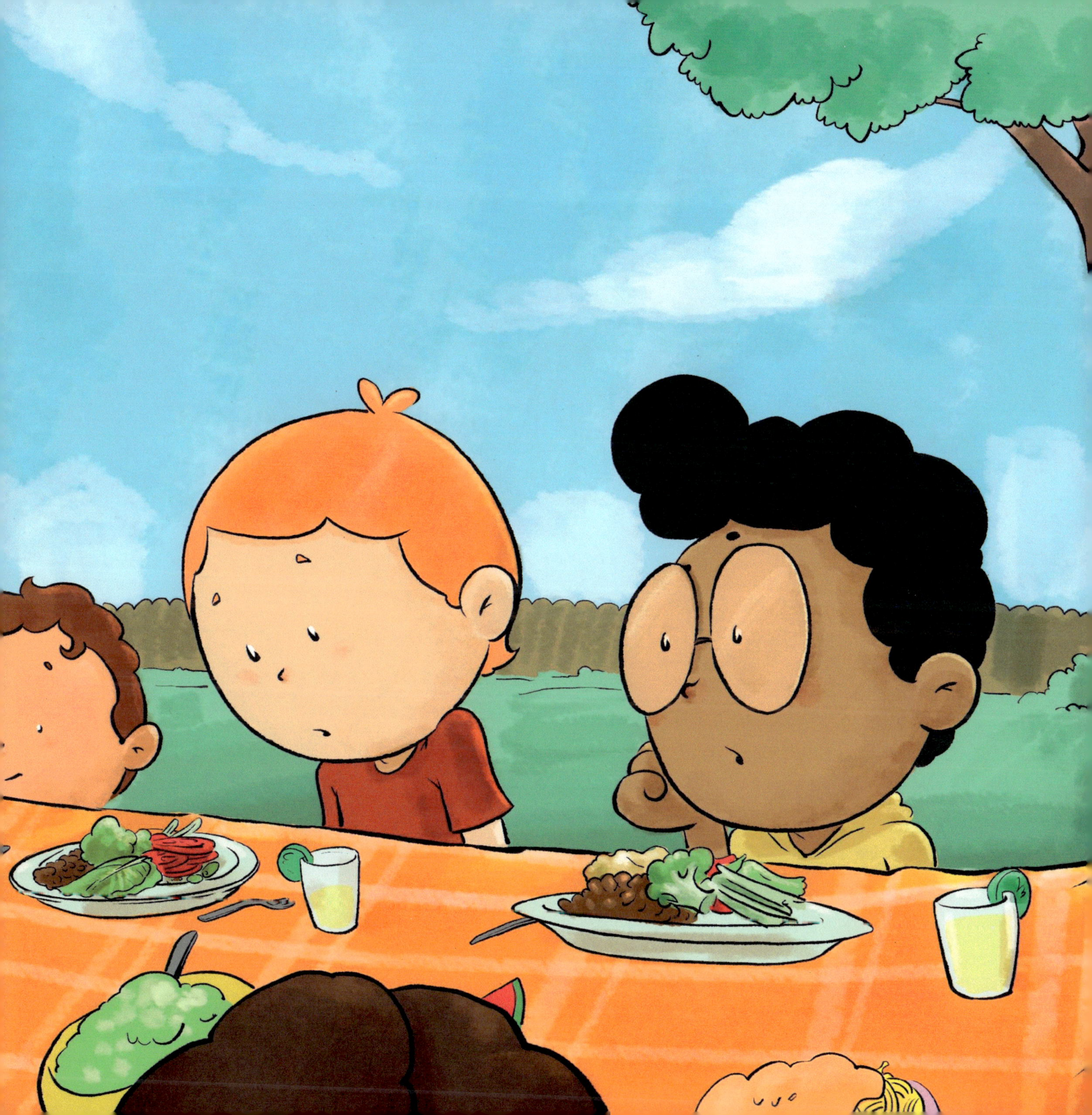

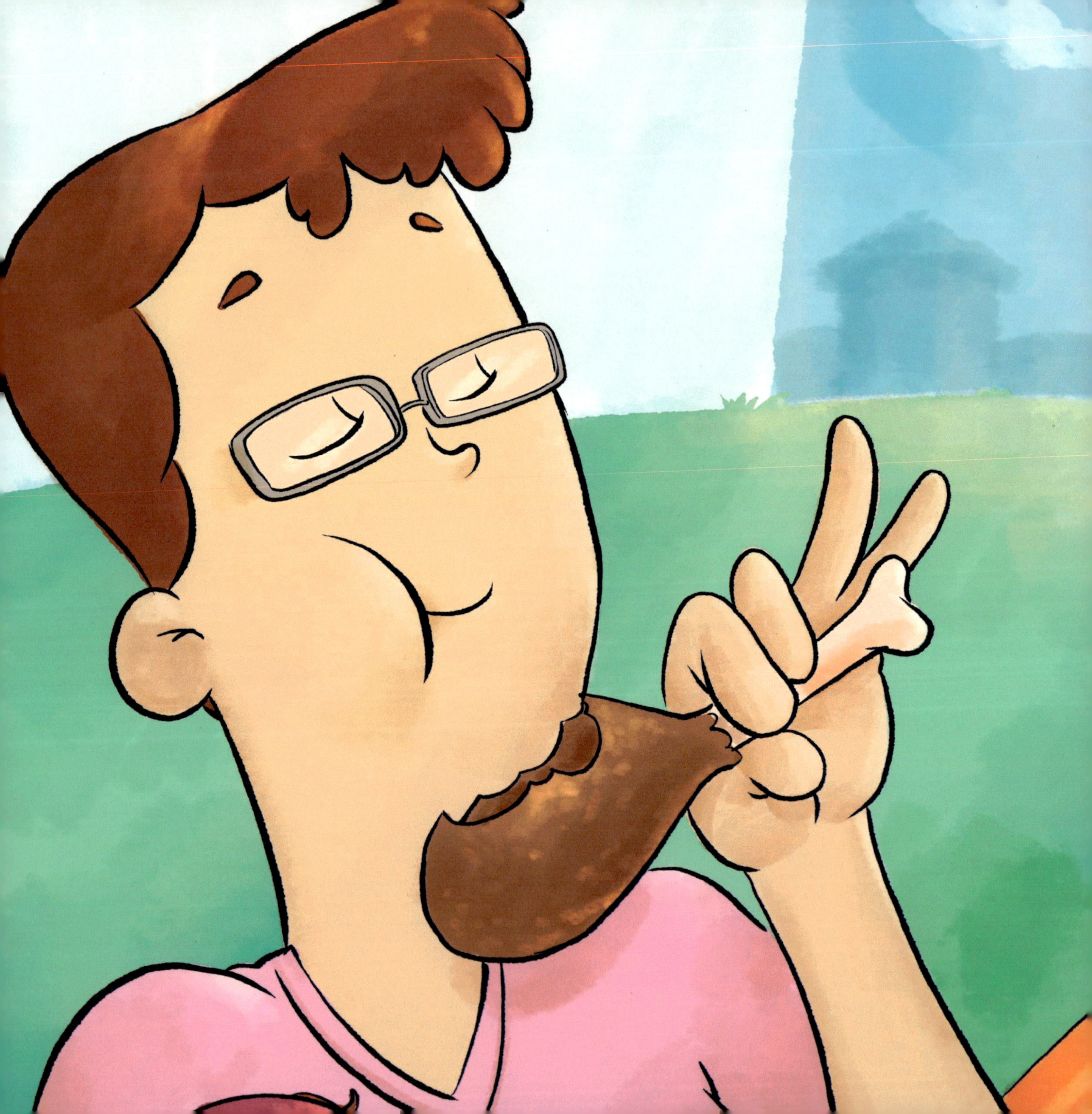

"WHAT IS THAT OVER THERE?", TO HIS MOM, ASKED BALOO.
"THAT IS CALLED MEAT BUT IT IS NOT FOR YOU."

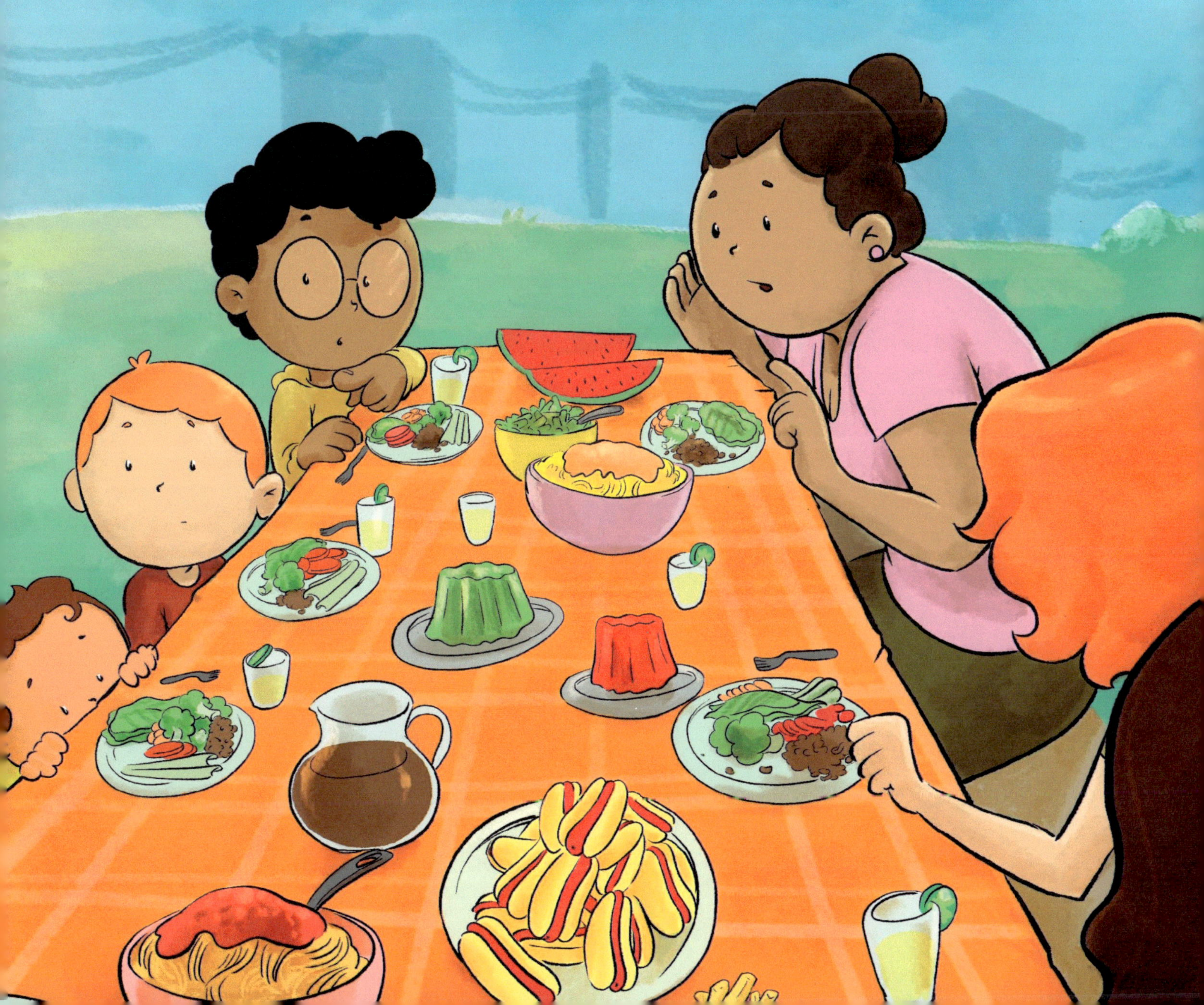

"THEY ARE EATING MEAT, DOES THAT MEAN THEY ARE BAD?"
"OF COURSE NOT, SON, BUT IT DOES MAKE ME SAD."

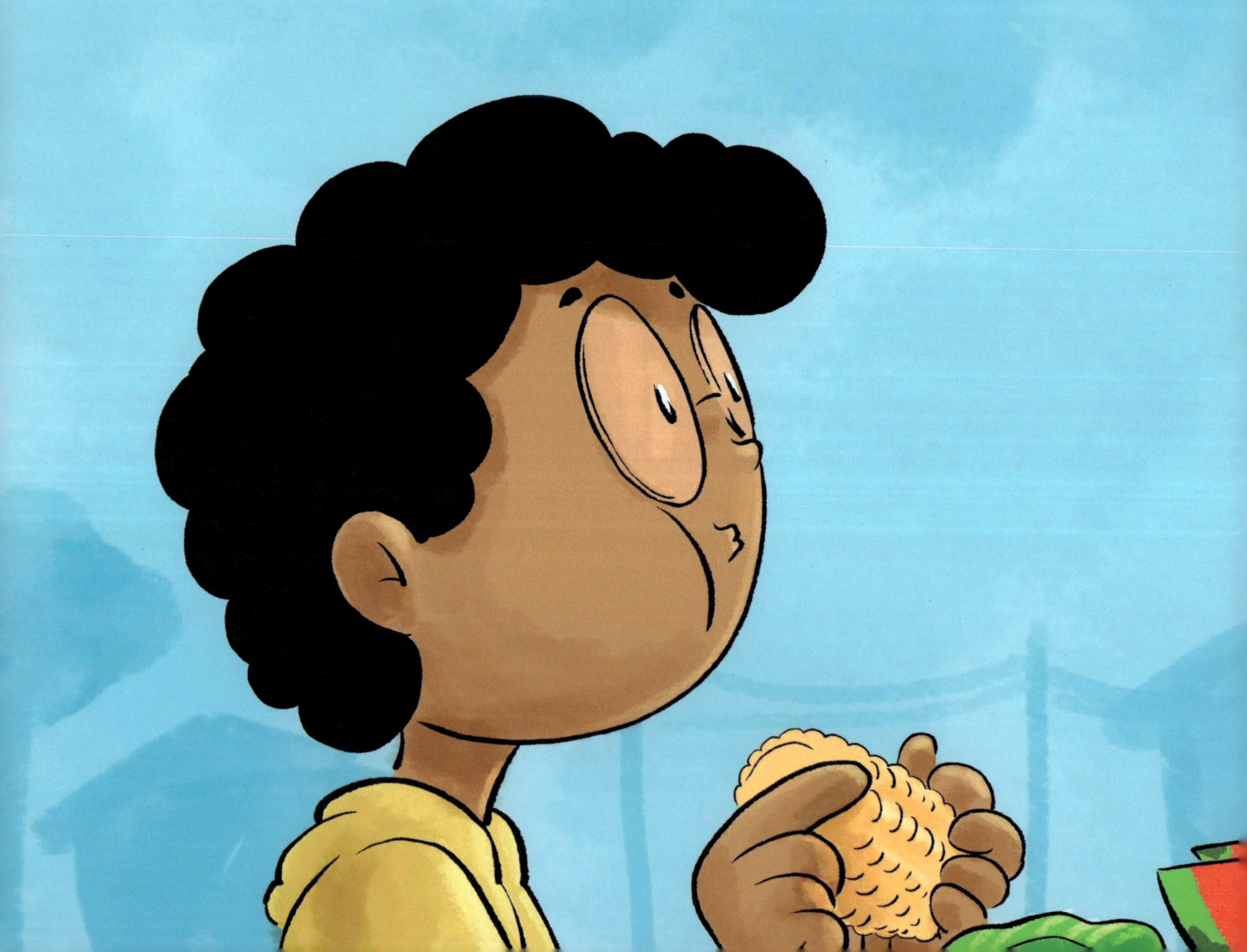

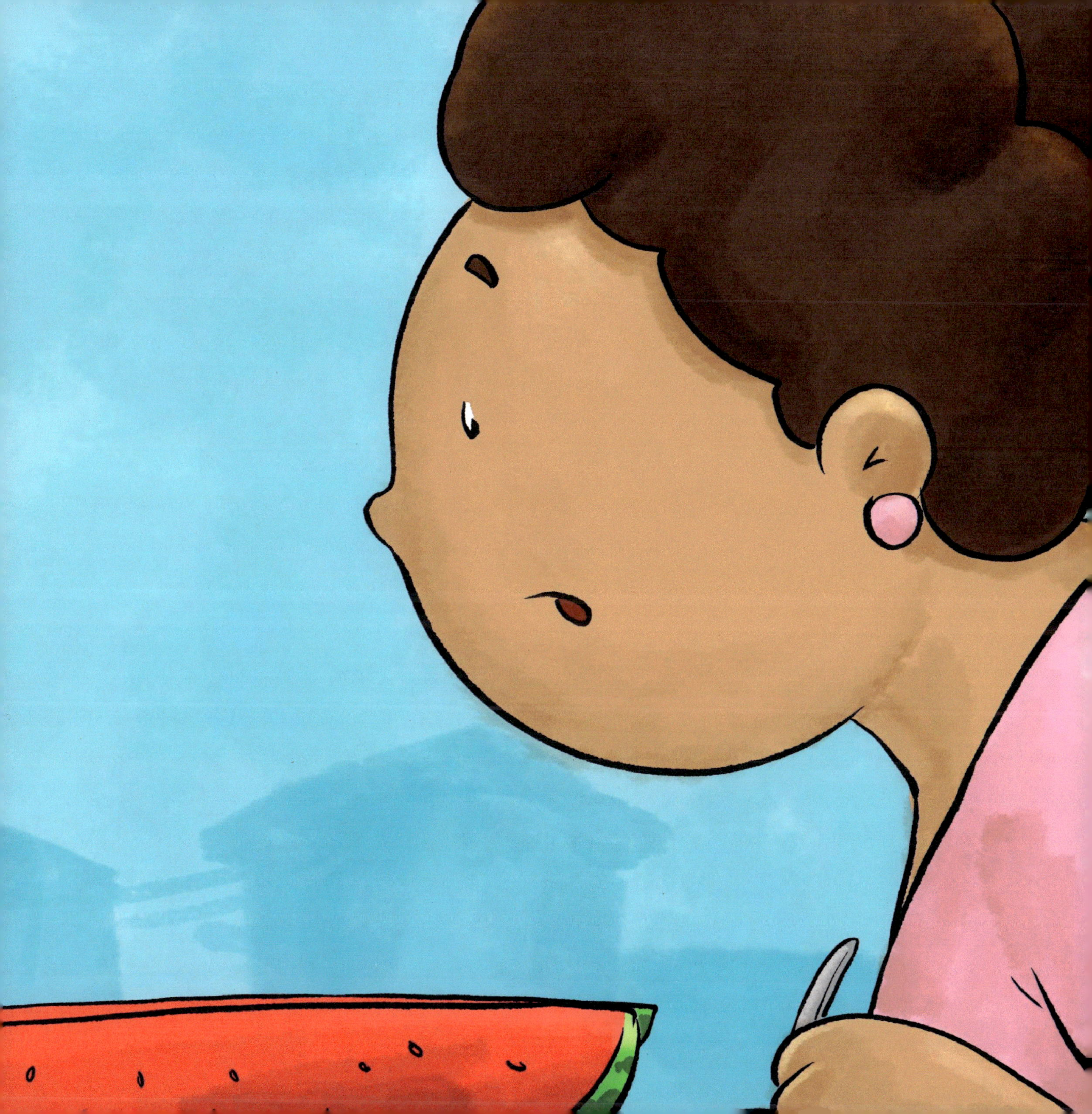

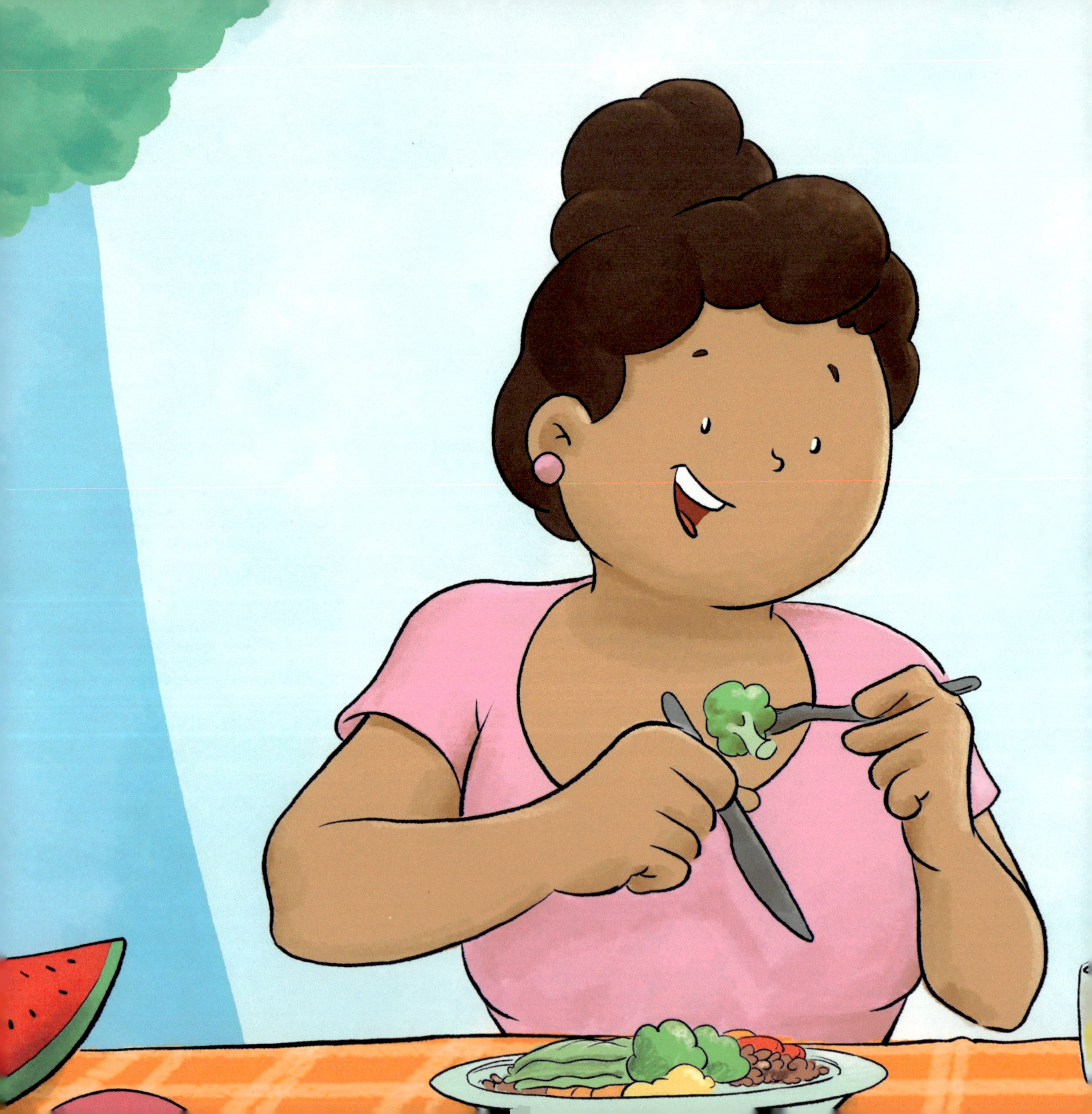

"MEAT IS MADE OF ANIMALS AND WE CHOOSE NOT TO PARTAKE,
BUT IT'S A PERSONAL CONVICTION THAT ONE HAS TO MAKE."

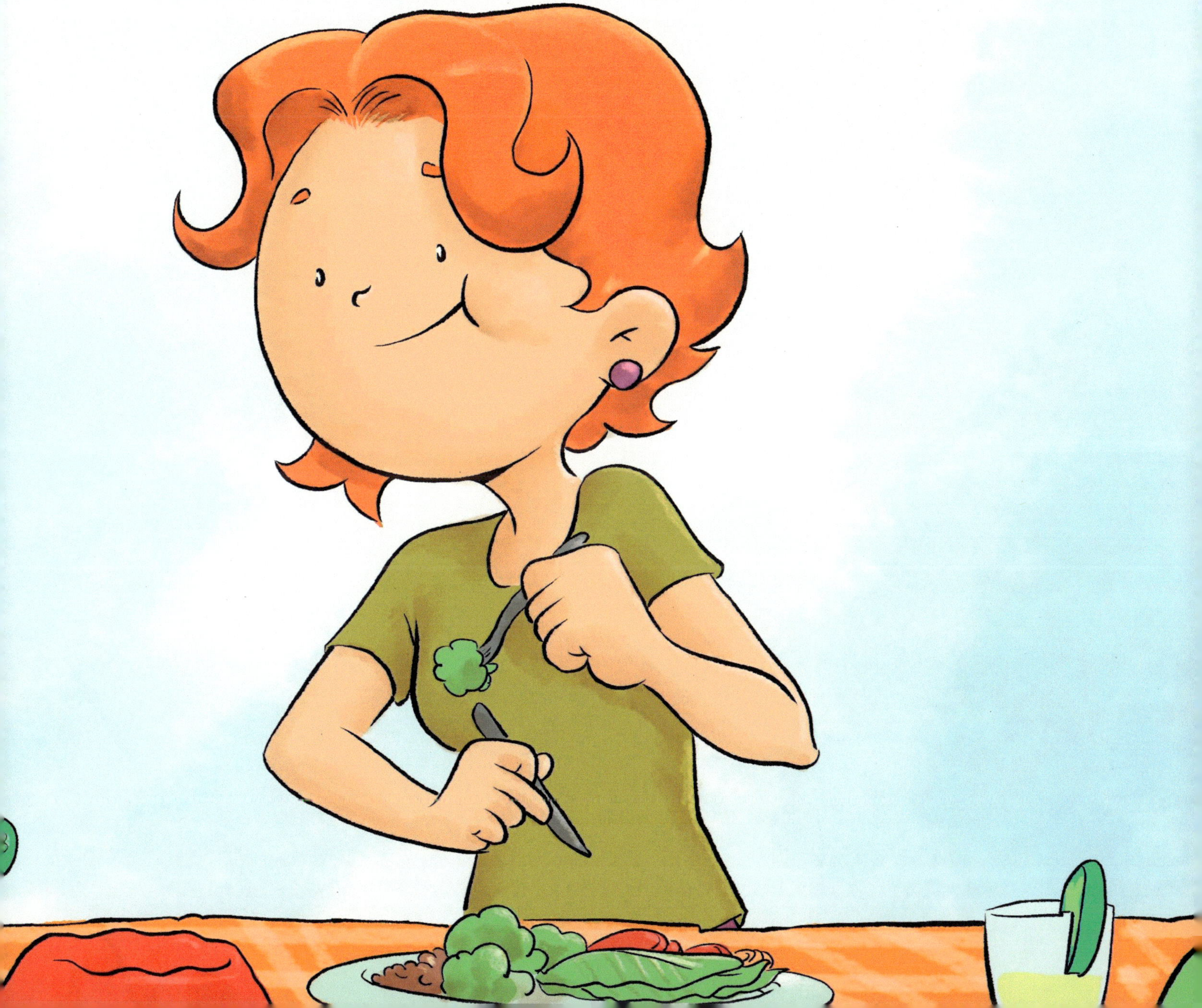

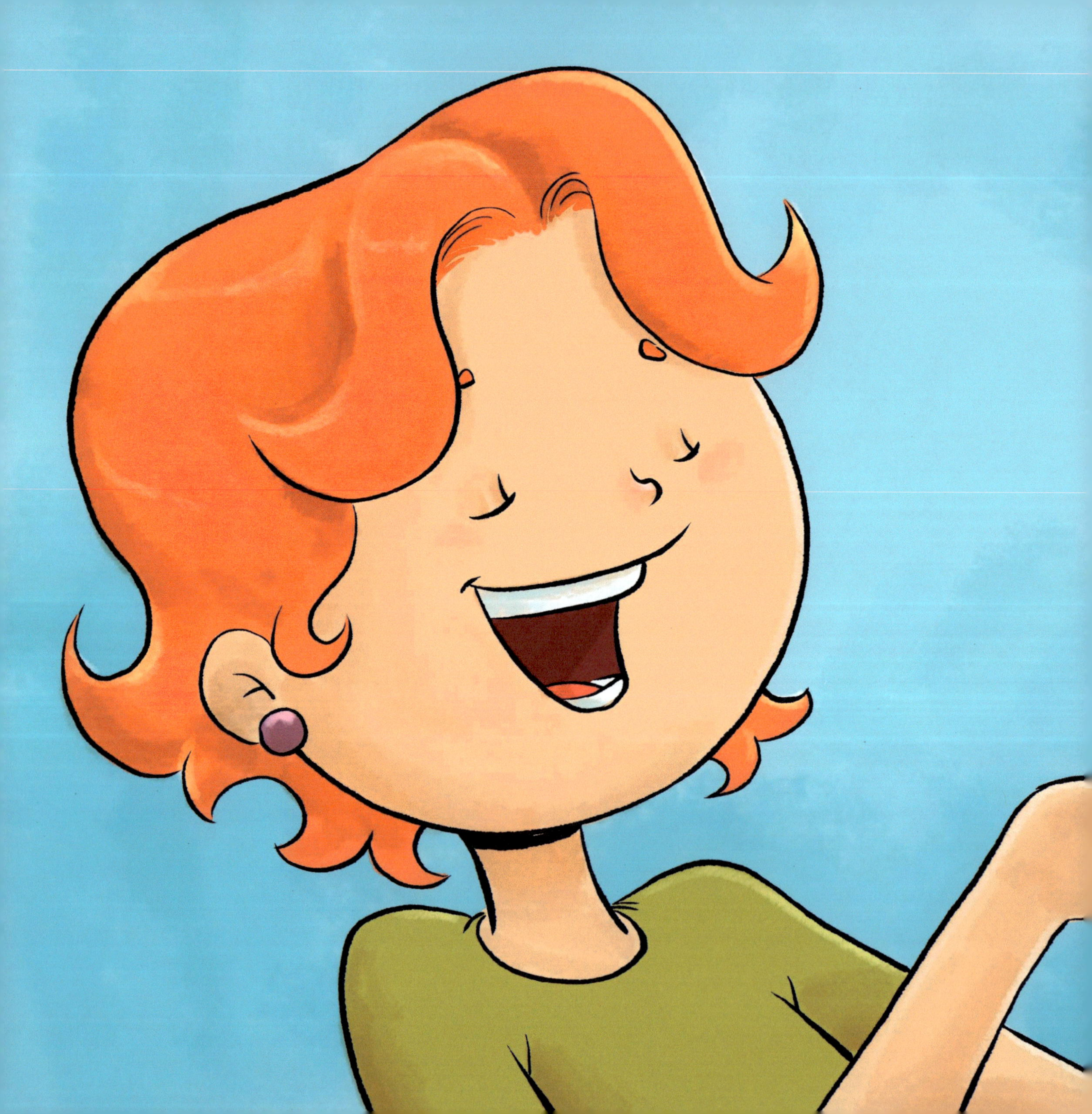

"DIFFERENT PEOPLE EAT DIFFERENT THINGS,
WE JUST CHOOSE TO EAT PLANTS BECAUSE IT MAKES OUR HEARTS SING."

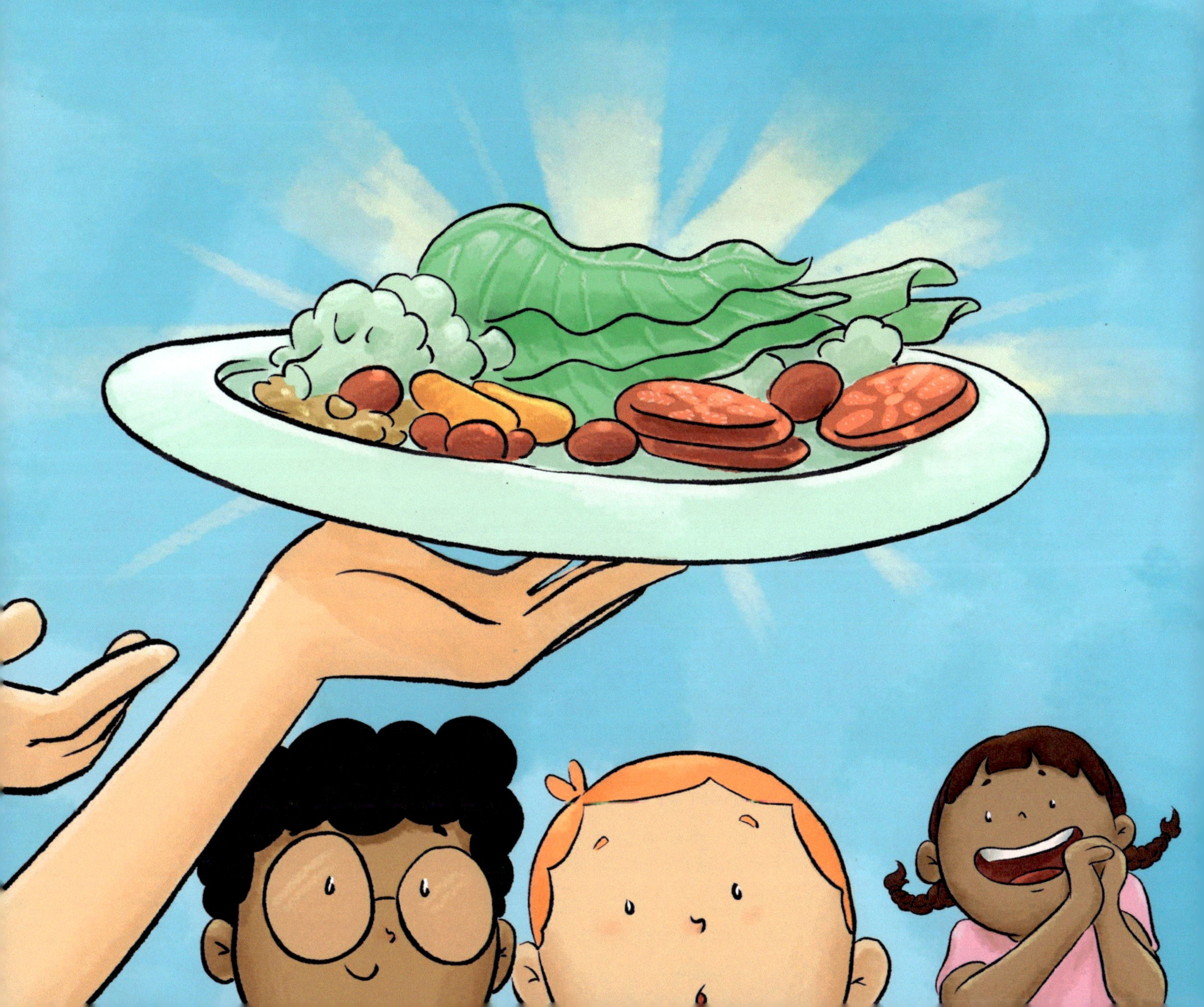

"SOME PEOPLE EAT MEAT AND SOME ONLY EAT FISH,
SOME WILL ONLY EAT EGGS AND CHEESE IN THEIR DISH."

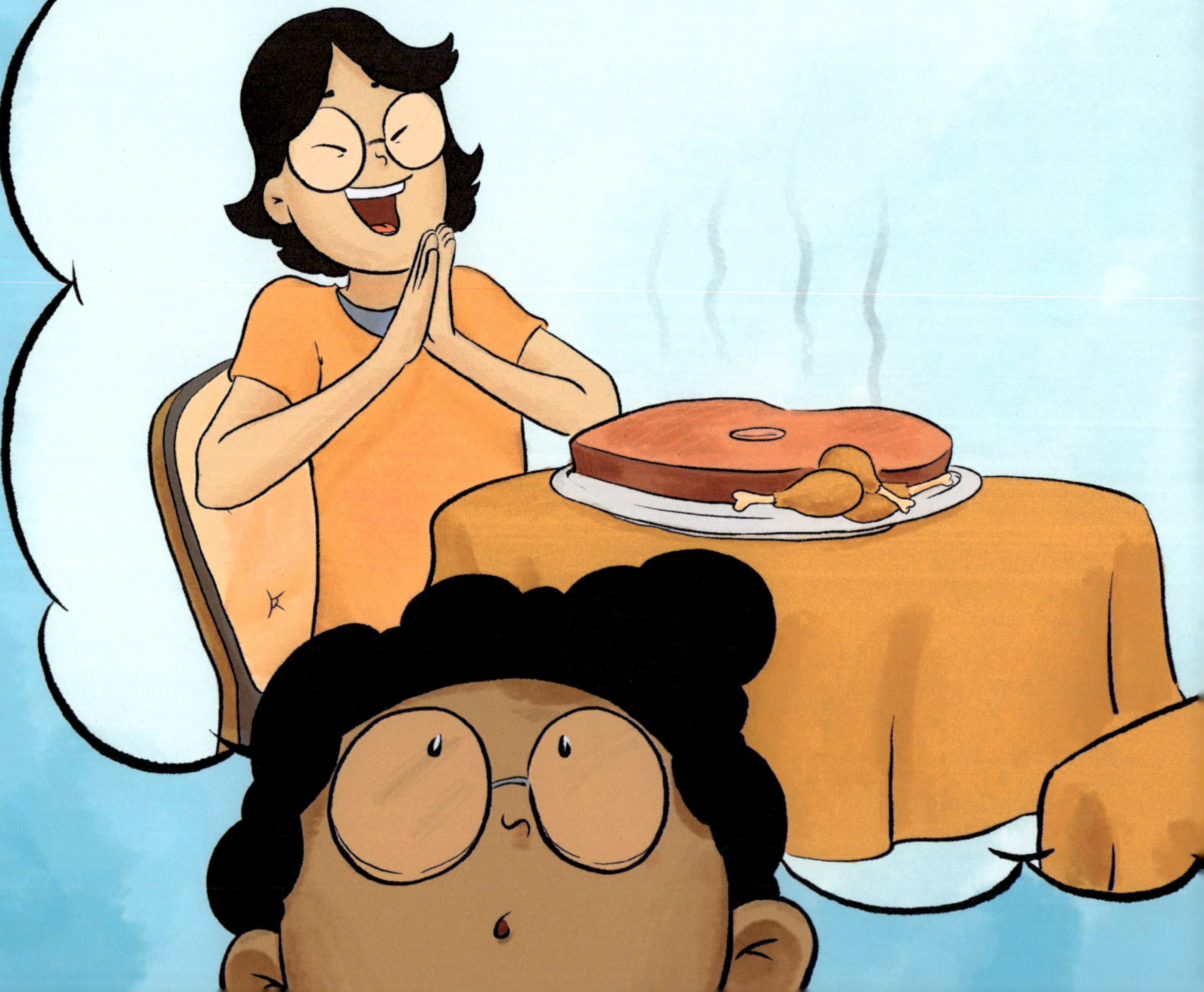

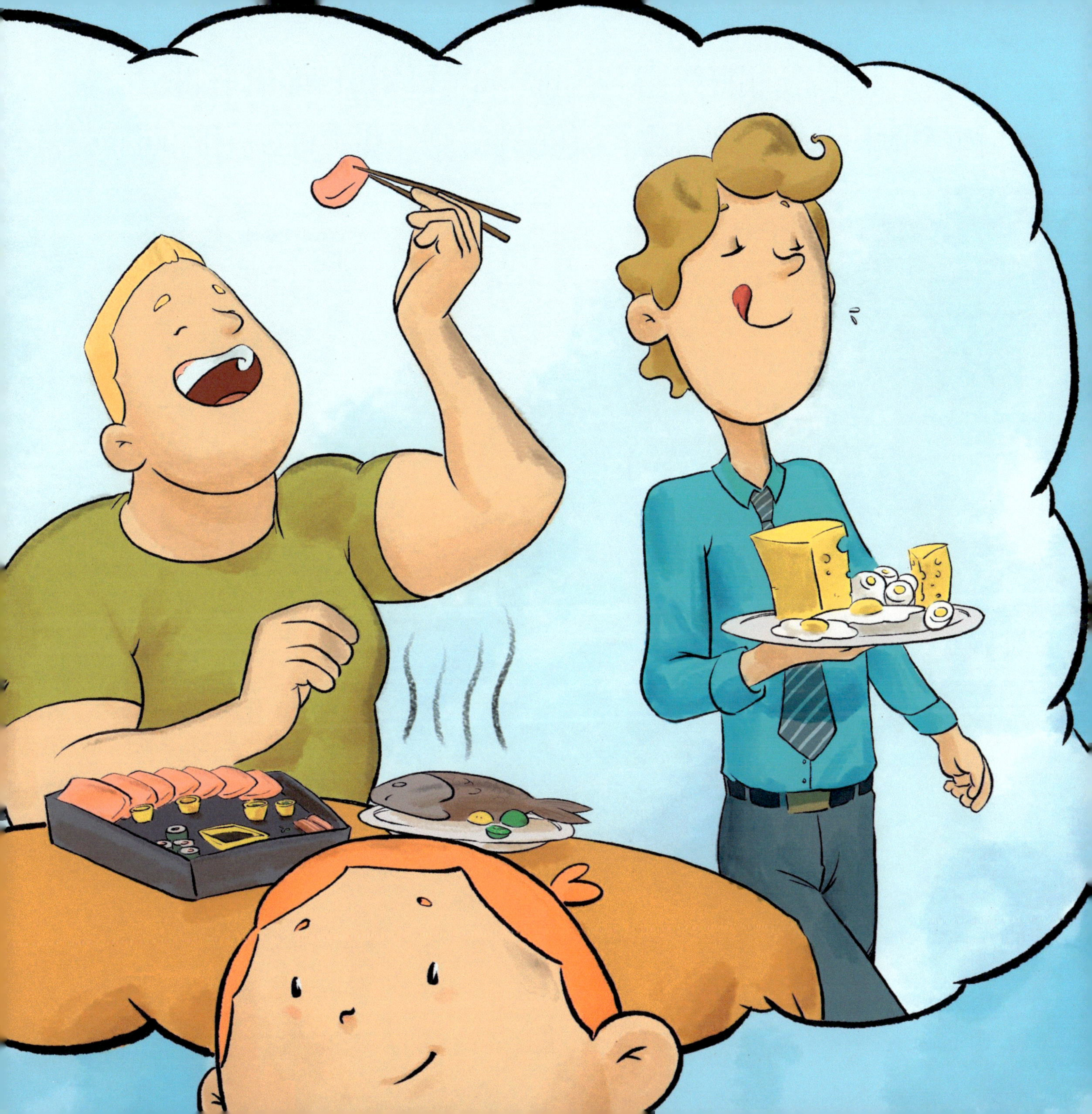

"THERE ARE OTHERS LIKE US THAT MOST ENJOY WHOLE FOODS BUT SOME FAMILIES PREFER THE CONVENIENCE OF A DRIVE-THROUGH."

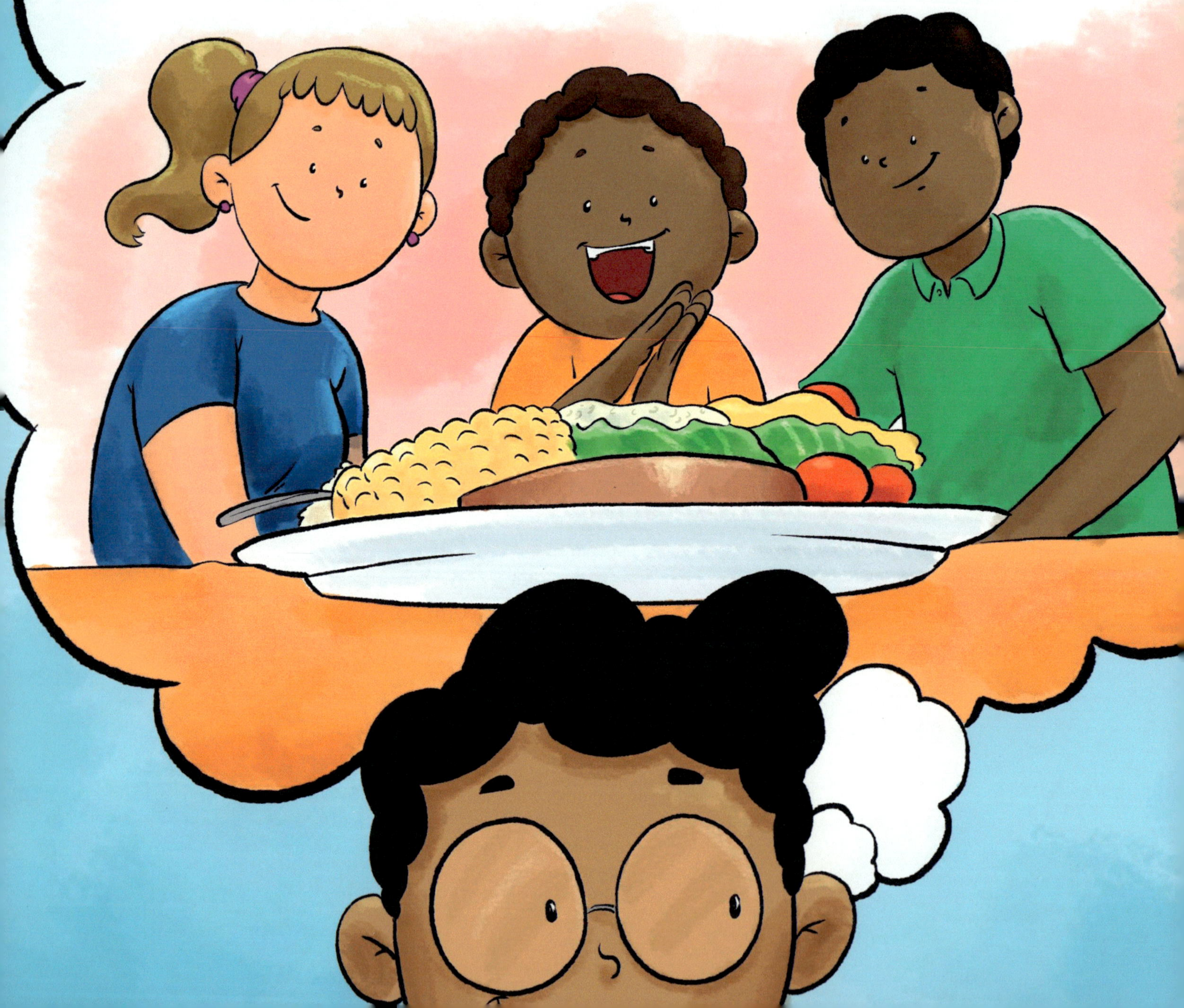

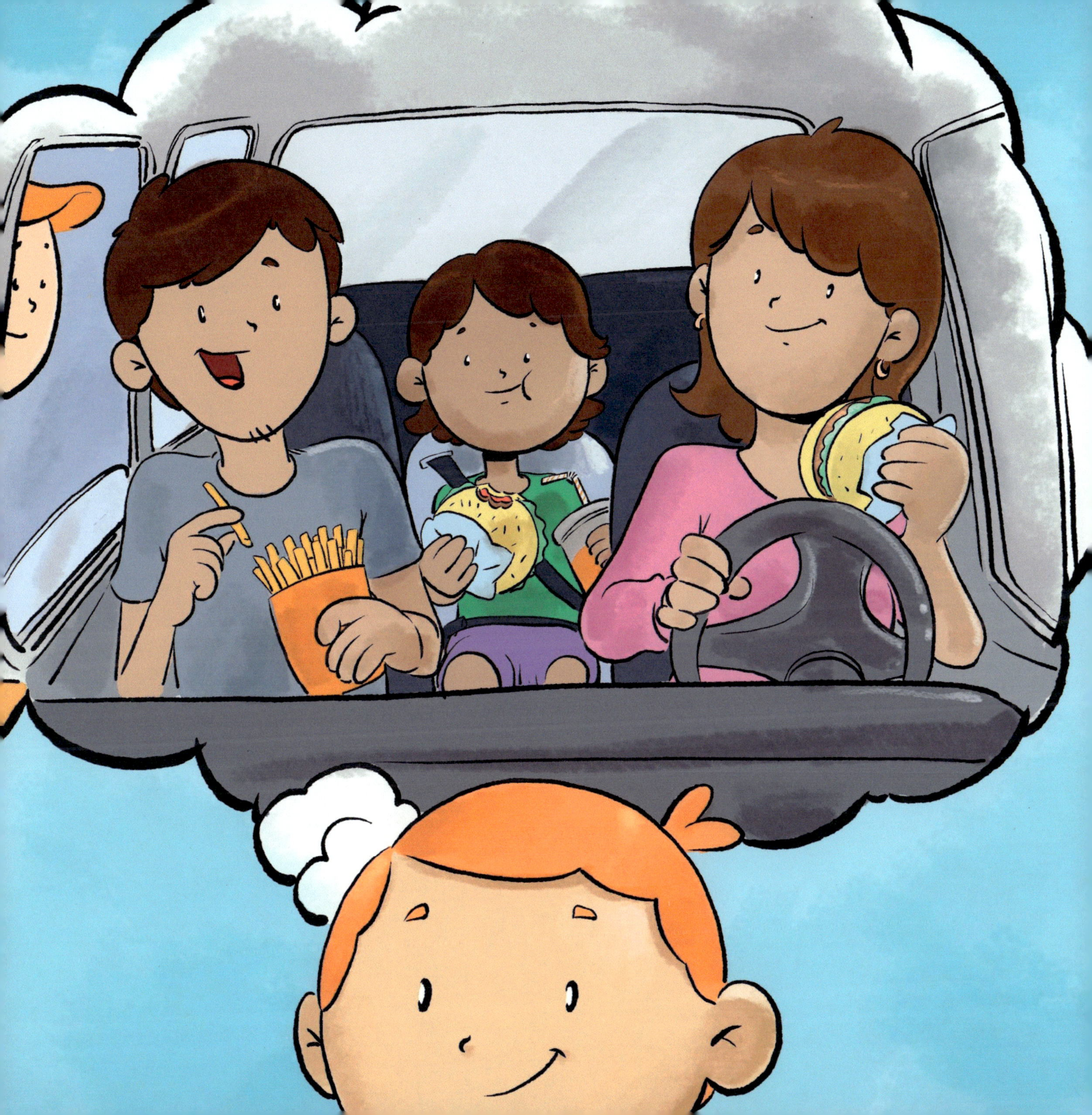

"EVERYONE HAS THEIR OWN SPECIAL DIET,
ONE DAY WHEN YOU'RE OLDER YOU MAY DECIDE TO TRY IT."

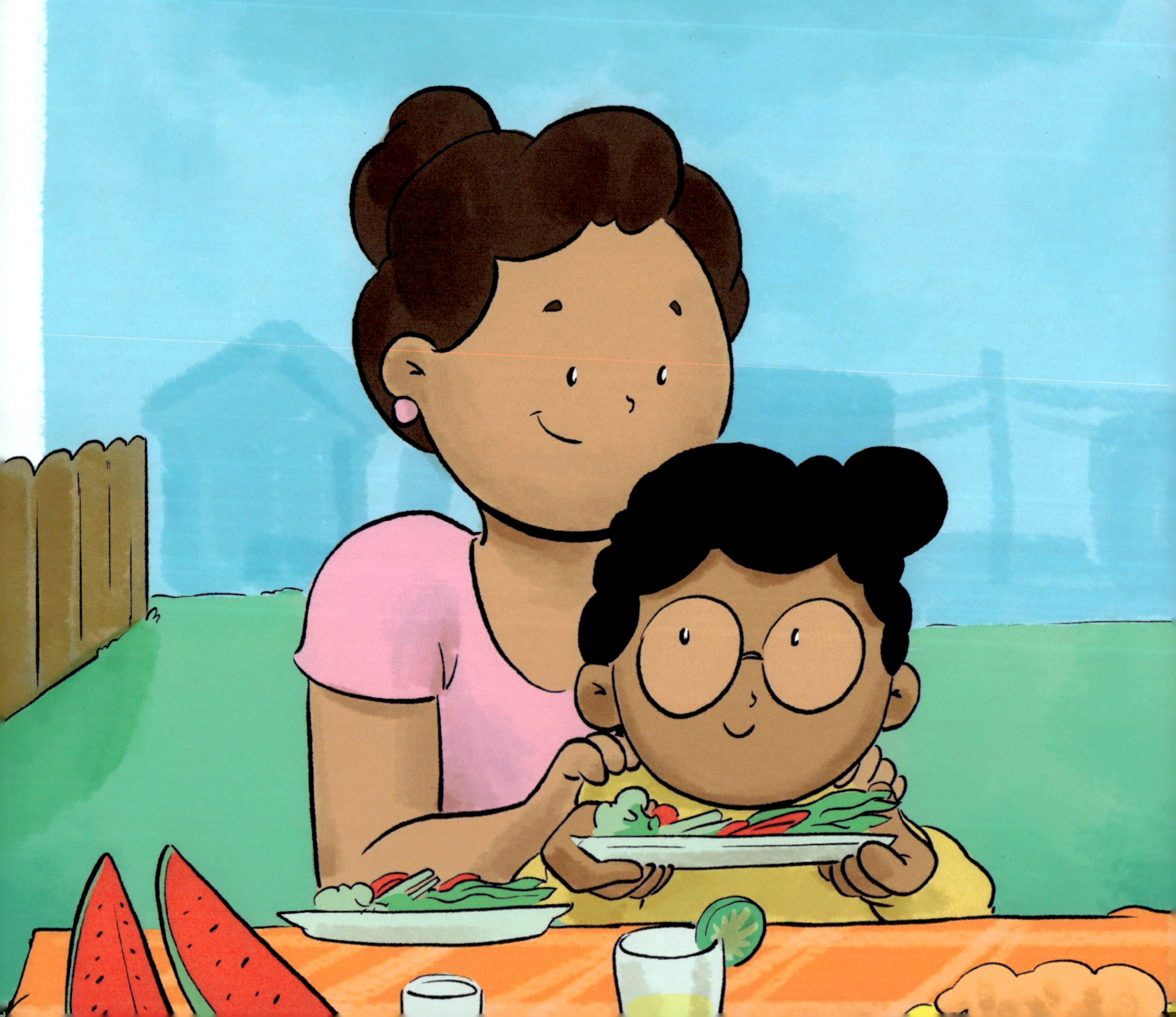

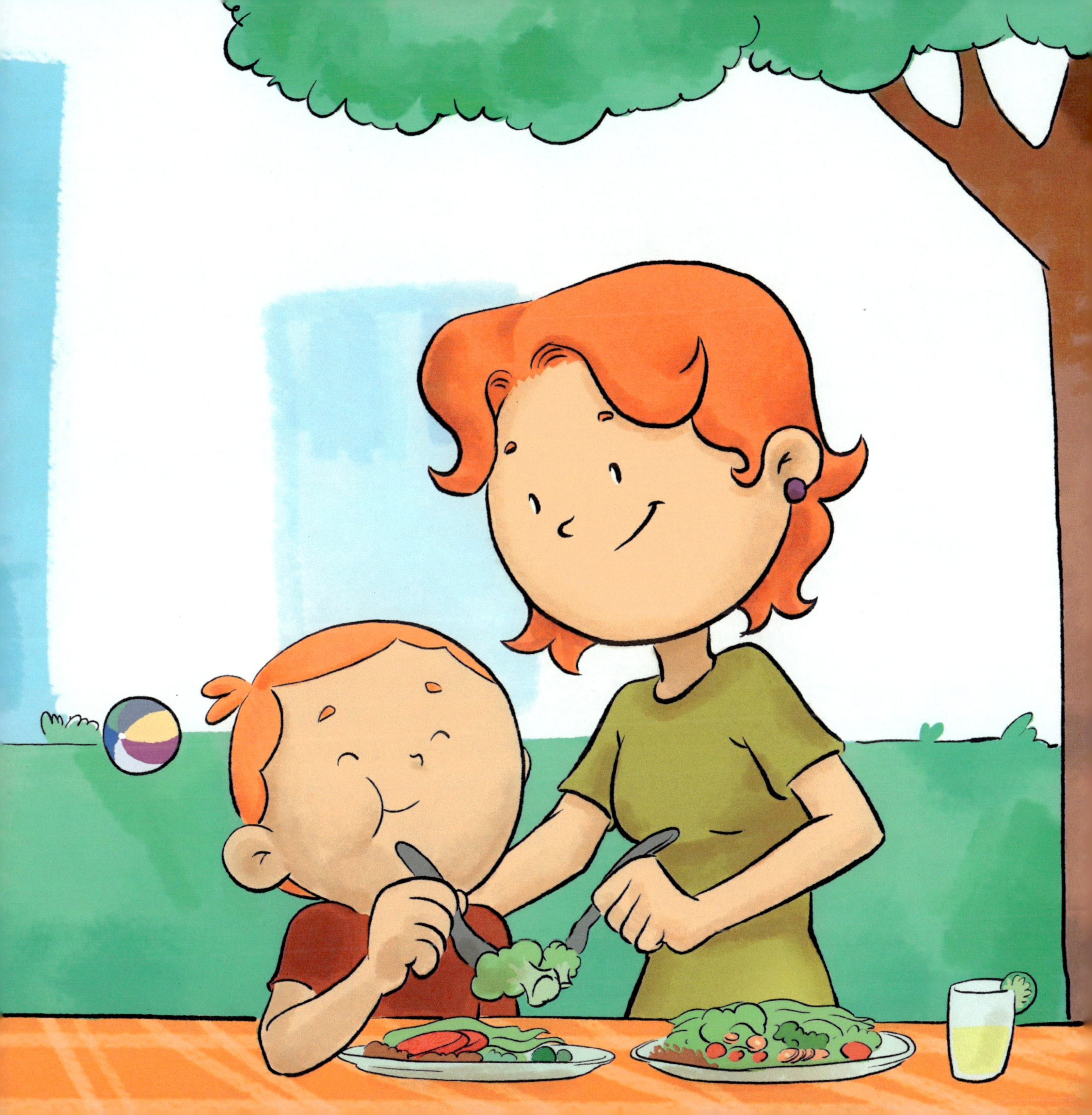

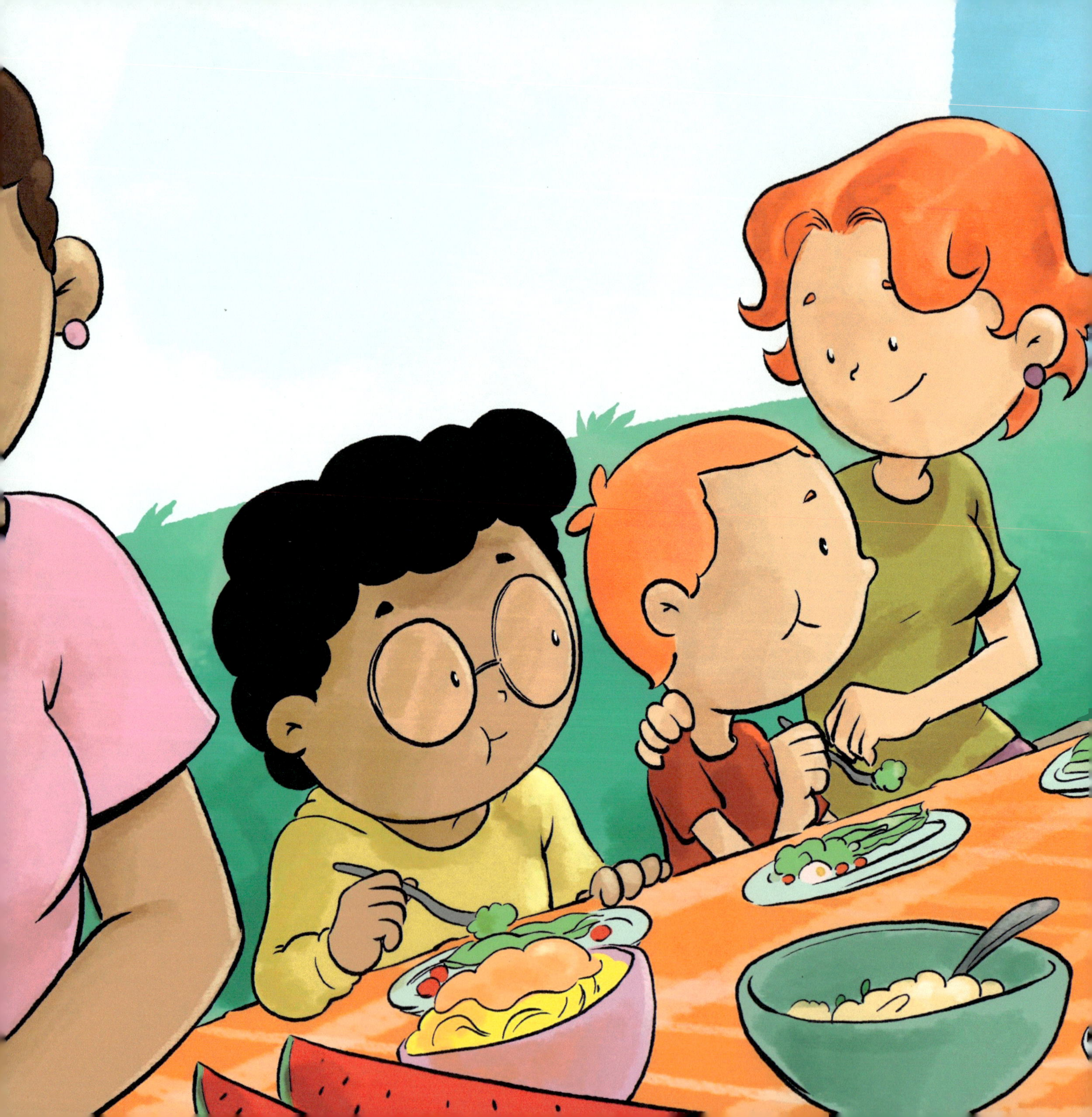

"YOU SHOULD BE FRIENDS WITH EVERYONE AND NOT FOCUS ON THEIR FOOD,
WE ALL NEED TO EAT, IT'S NOT WORTH A FEUD."

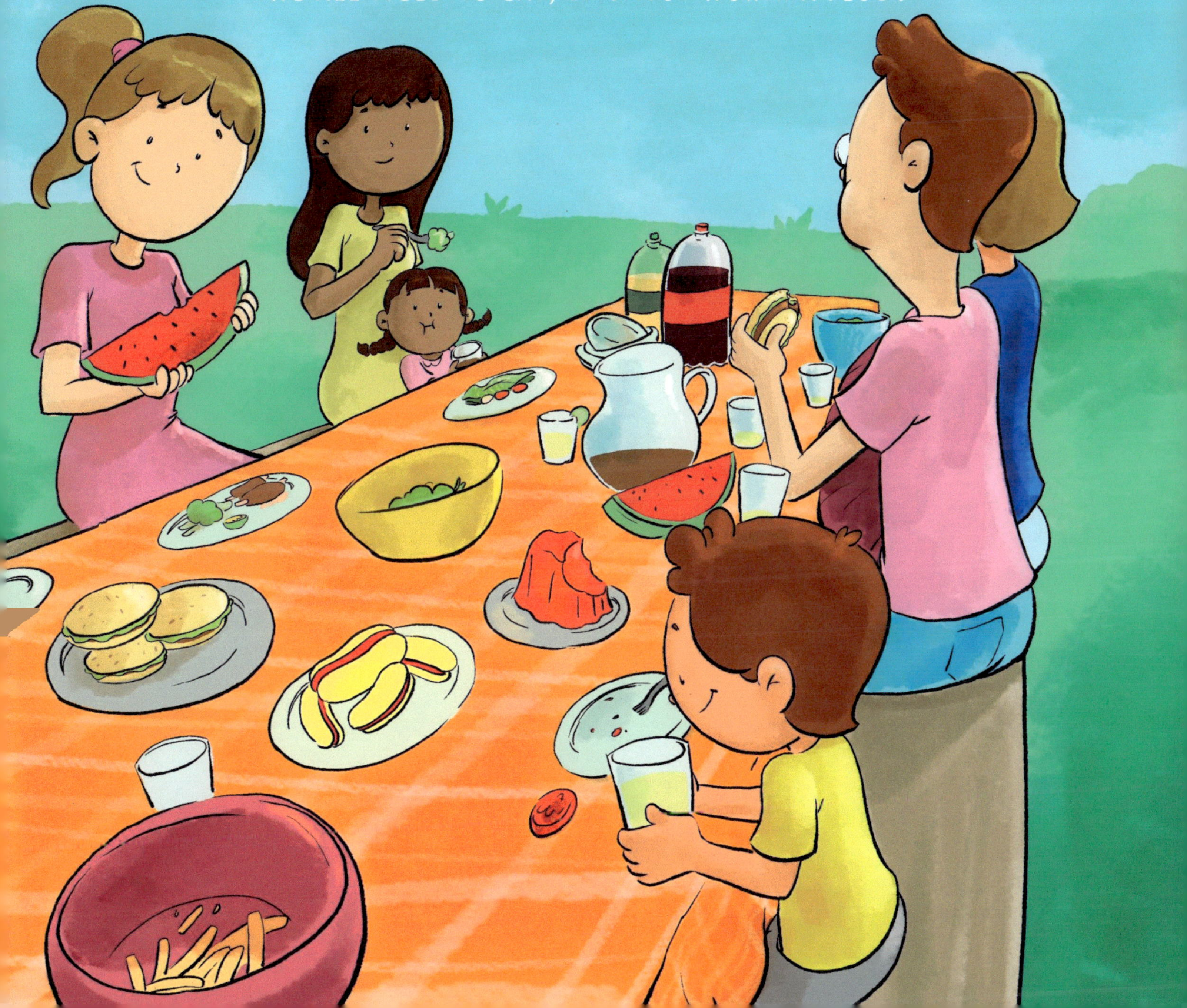

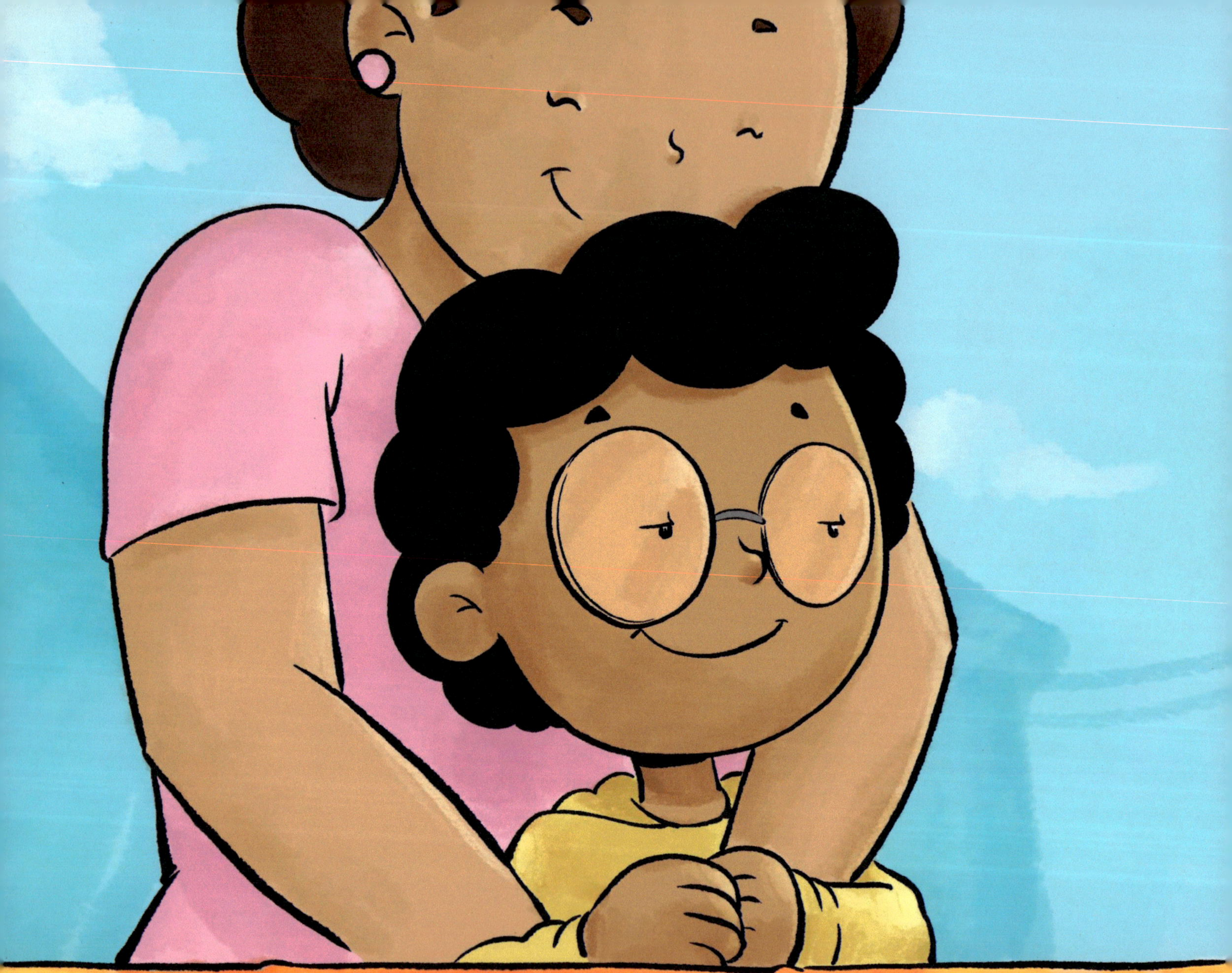

BALOO SMILED AT MAZE AND THEY FINISHED THEIR PLATES,
NO LONGER THINKING ABOUT WHAT EVERYONE ATE.

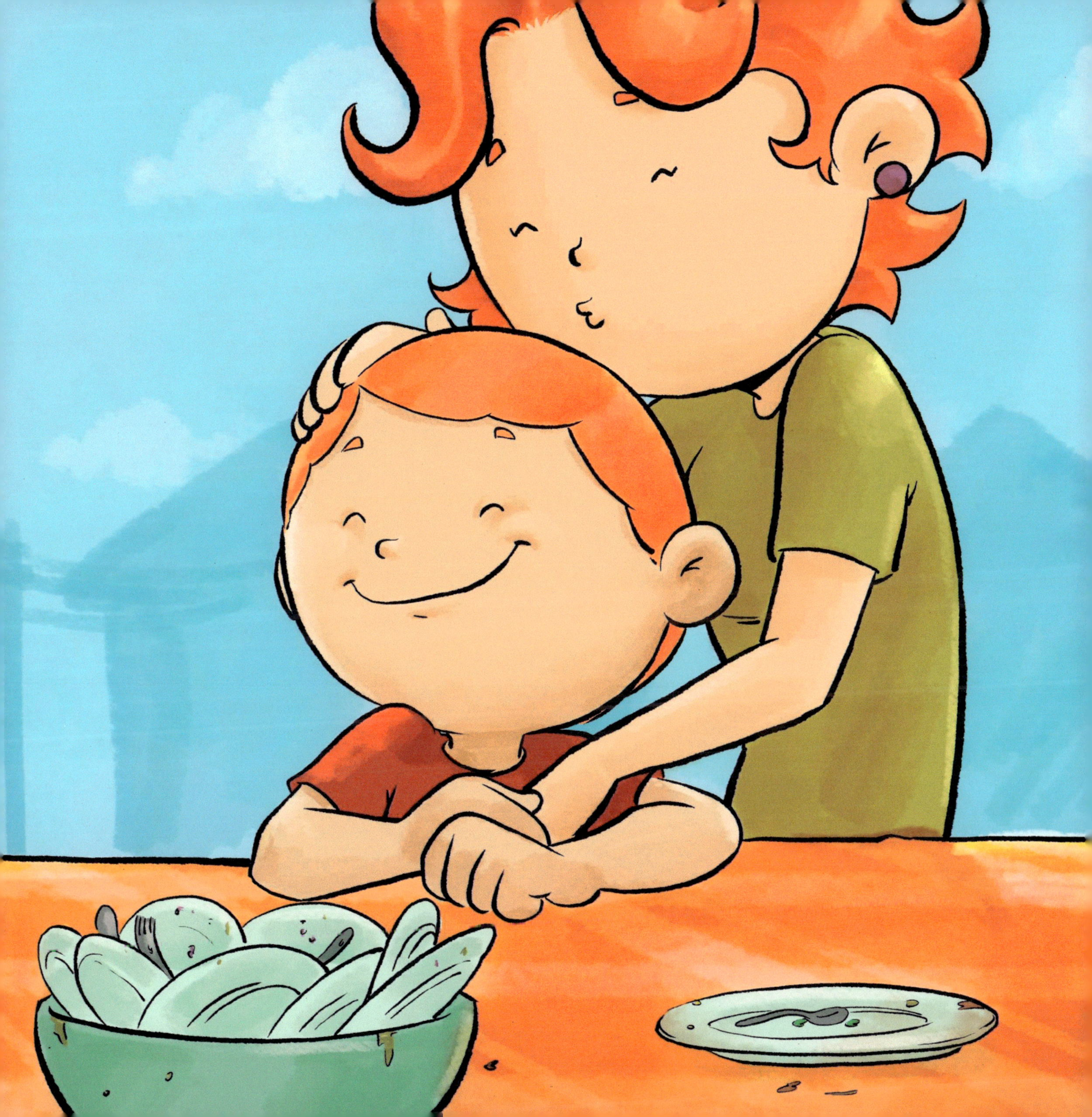

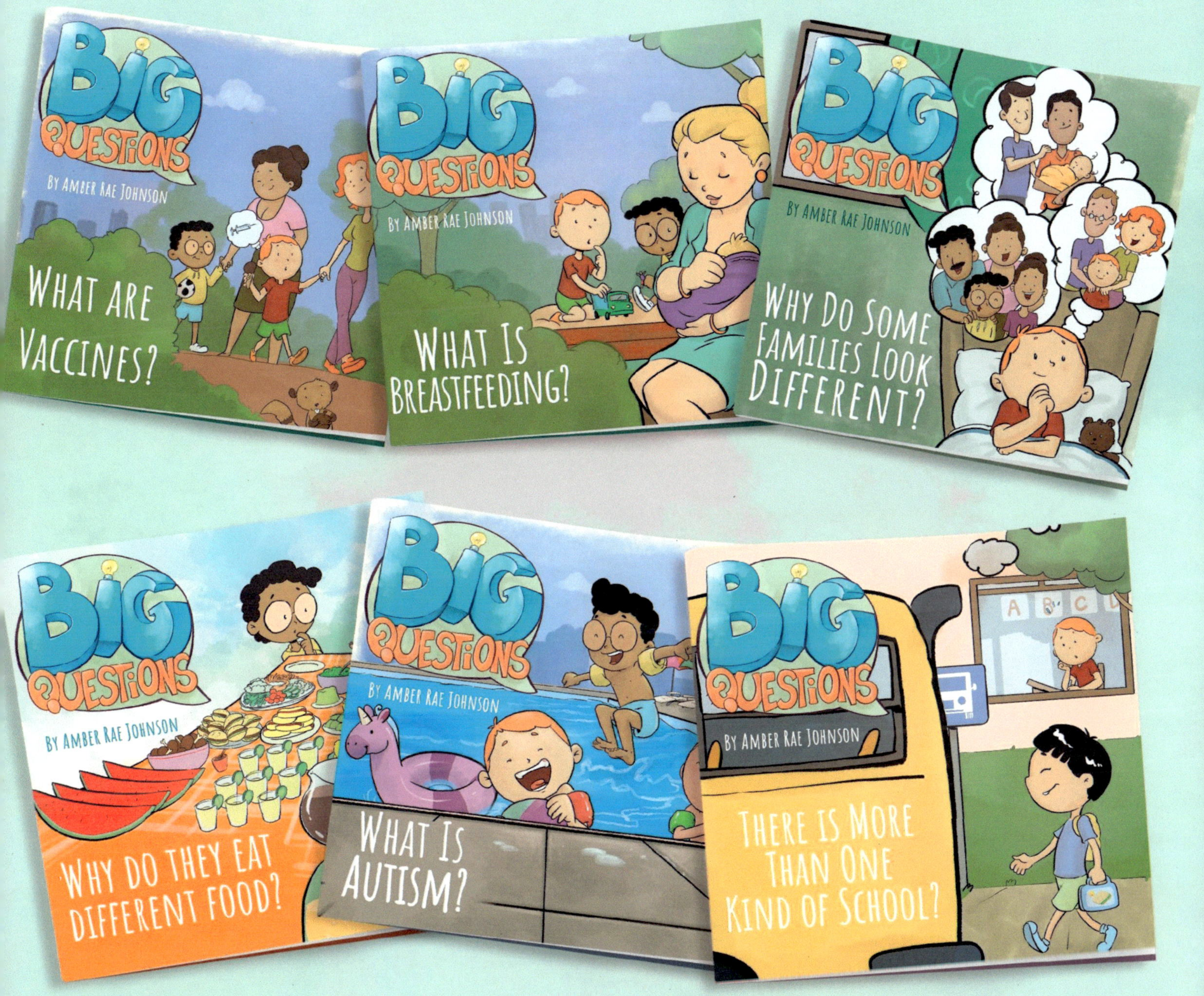

@BIGQUESTIONSBOOKS @BQBOOKS @BIGQUESTIONSBOOKS

Connect the dots on the picnic basket!

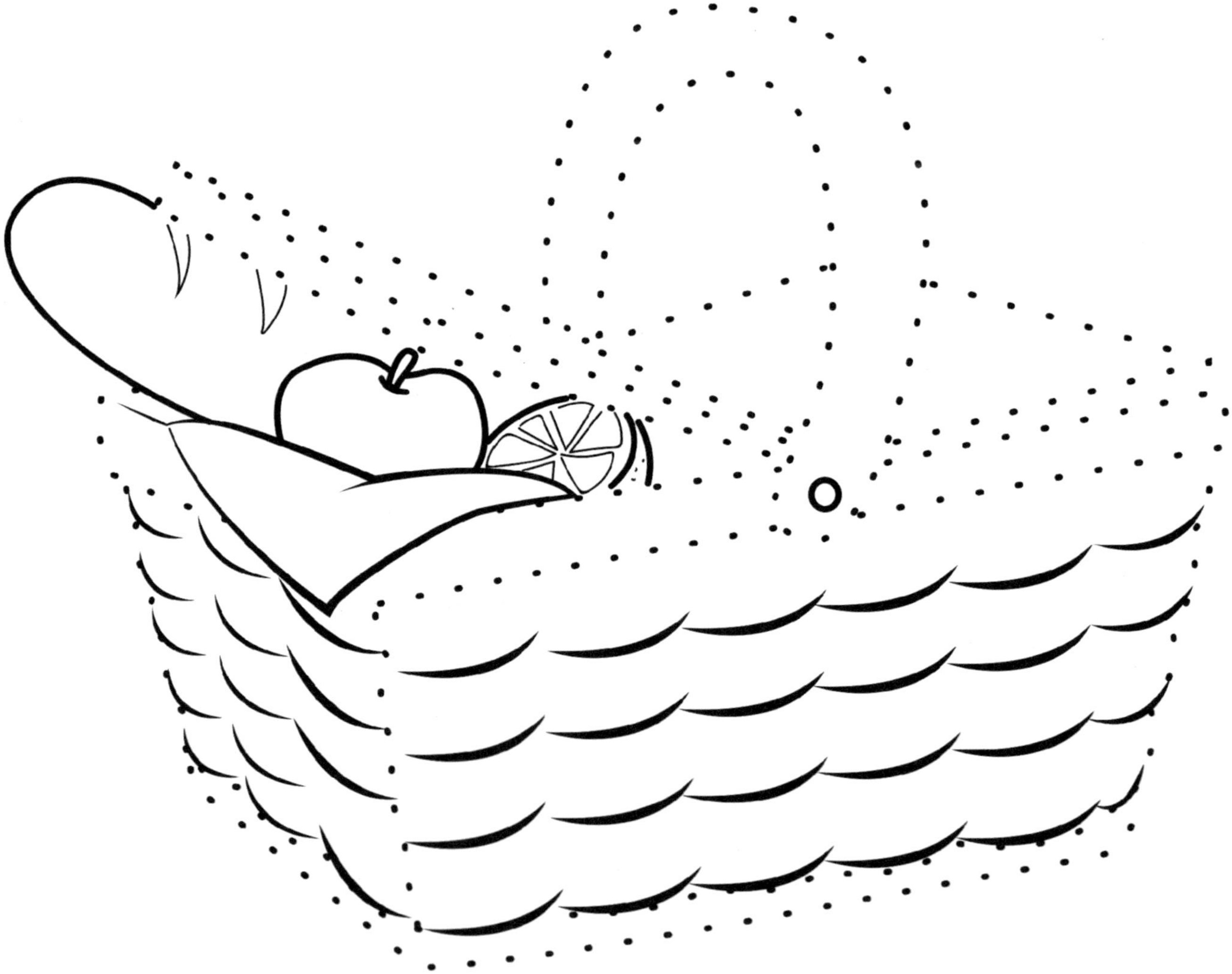

COLOR TIME!

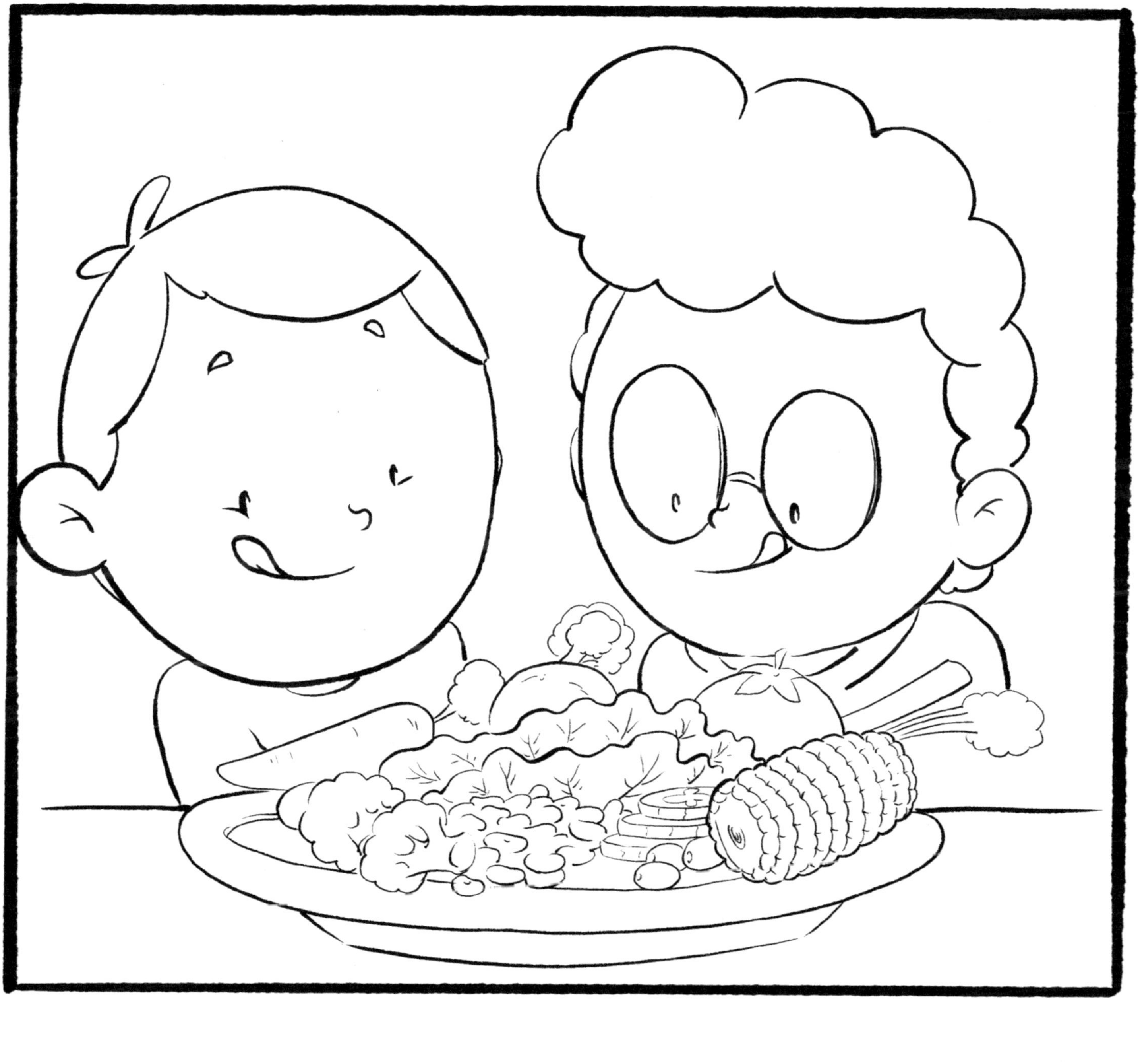

Made in United States
Troutdale, OR
11/03/2026

56844877R00024